CHEMICAL PEELS

Step by Step®
CHEMICAL PEELS

Second Edition

Editor

Niti Khunger MD DDV DNB
Professor and Consultant Dermatologist
Department of Dermatology and STD
Vardhman Mahavir Medical College and
Safdarjung Hospital
New Delhi, India

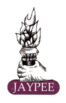

JAYPEE

JAYPEE BROTHERS MEDICAL PUBLISHERS (P) LTD
New Delhi • London • Philadelphia • Panama

Jaypee Brothers Medical Publishers (P) Ltd

Headquarters
Jaypee Brothers Medical Publishers (P) Ltd
4838/24, Ansari Road, Daryaganj
New Delhi 110 002, India
Phone: +91-11-43574357
Fax: +91-11-43574314
Email: jaypee@jaypeebrothers.com

Overseas Offices
J.P. Medical Ltd.
83, Victoria Street, London
SW1H 0HW (UK)
Phone: +44-2031708910
Fax: +02-03-0086180
Email: info@jpmedpub.com

Jaypee Medical Inc.
The Bourse
111, South Independence Mall East
Suite 835, Philadelphia, PA 19106, USA
Phone: +1 267-519-9789
Email: jpmed.us@jaypeebrothers.com

Jaypee Brothers Medical Publishers (P) Ltd.
Bhotahity, Kathmandu, Nepal
Phone: +977-9741283608
Email: kathmandu@jaypeebrothers.com

Jaypee-Highlights Medical Publishers Inc.
City of Knowledge, Bld. 237, Clayton
Panama City, Panama
Phone: +1 507-301-0496
Fax: +1 507-301-0499
Email: cservice@jphmedical.com

Jaypee Brothers Medical Publishers (P) Ltd.
17/1-B, Babar Road, Block-B, Shaymali
Mohammadpur, Dhaka-1207
Bangladesh
Mobile: +08801912003485
Email: jaypeedhaka@gmail.com

Website: www.jaypeebrothers.com
Website: www.jaypeedigital.com

© 2014, Jaypee Brothers Medical Publishers

Inquiries for bulk sales may be solicited at: jaypee@jaypeebrothers.com

Step by Step® Chemical Peels

First Edition: 2009

Second Edition: **2014**

ISBN: 978-93-5152-311-6

Printed at: Samrat Offset Pvt. Ltd.

Dedicated to

All my patients
who inspire me to
Innovate, Improvise and Implement

To my family
Drs Jitender, Monica and Arjun
who encourage me to
Aspire, Ascend and Achieve

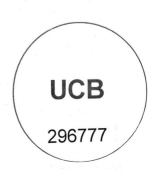

Contributors

Amar Vedamurthy MBBS
Resident Physician
Mount Auburn Hospital, USA
330, Mt. Auburn, St. Cambridge
MA 02138, USA
Harvard Medical School
25, Shattuck Street Boston
MA 02115, USA

Jaishree Sharad MD
CEO and Consultant Cosmetic Dermatologist
Skinfinite Aesthetic
Skin and Laser Clinic
Mumbai, Maharashtra, India

Maya Vedamurthy MD FRCP (Edin)
Dermatologist
RSV Skin and Laser Centre
Mahalingapuram, Chennai, Tamil Nadu, India

Monica Khunger MBBS
Resident
All India Institute of Medical Sciences
New Delhi, India

Niti Khunger MD DDV DNB
Professor and Consultant Dermatologist
Department of Dermatology and STD
Vardhman Mahavir Medical College and
Safdarjung Hospital
New Delhi, India

Shenaz Arsiwala MD
Consultant Dermatologist
Cosmetologist and Dermatosurgeon
Saifee Hospital and Prince Aly Khan Hospital
Mumbai, Maharashtra, India

Preface to the Second Edition

The overwhelming response of the first edition compelled me to bring the second edition. Three new chapters have been added on chemical peeling in acne and acne scars, facial melanoses and periocular peels. There is a definite place for chemical peels in active acne, particularly in comedonal acne, pustular acne and acne with pigmentation. The focus of the chapter on facial melanoses is on selecting the right peel in darker skin types. The response in darker skins can be unpredictable and an inappropriate peel can lead to aggravation of the pigmentation. The chapter on periocular peels highlights the special considerations when peeling the sensitive periocular region. Modification of standard techniques can make this area safer to peel.

The popularity of the previous edition was based on the practical readability, cookbook approach and convenient pocket size of the book. This format has been retained at the cost of repetition, to make the book a handy reference for a busy practitioner in the clinic as well as a fresh physician beginning a career in chemical peels.

Niti Khunger

Preface to the First Edition

Chemical peeling is an ancient procedure that has stood the test of time for rejuvenating the skin. It is the application of a chemical agent of defined strength to the skin that causes destruction at the required depth, followed by remodeling without scarring.

In recent times, there has been an explosive interest in procedural techniques for skin rejuvenation and the trend is increasingly for procedures that are noninvasive or minimally invasive, requiring little downtime. The majority of the chemical peeling procedures fit into this category. The long-term experience with chemical peels has shown them to be safe and effective for a variety of common conditions like dyschromias, photoaging and acne. An added advantage is the relative low cost of these procedures as compared to lasers and other procedures to rejuvenate the skin. Lasers are still very expensive to acquire and maintain. This has led to a resurgence in the use of chemical peels, which is now a re-emerging art with newer peels and newer combinations.

New advances in peel approaches including combination, sequential and segmental peels are safer and lower-strength peeling agents are allowing clinicians to tailor their practices to patients' needs, often without added costs. Chemical peels are thus not only a part of the cosmetic scene of the past, but also a definite cornerstone of the future.

This book is a step-by-step practical guide to perform chemical peels. There is some repetition of the basic procedure in the chapters with the aim that the reader will find easier to follow, while doing a particular peel and not miss any important step. The interesting cases give examples of treatment in difficult situations, while ten golden rules summarize the essence of chemical peeling.

The aim of the book is to expose young physicians to the array of chemical peels available today and guide the practicing dermatologists how to safely use this versatile technique in the treatment of common day-to-day conditions such as skin rejuvenation, photoaging, melasma and acne.

Niti Khunger

Acknowledgments

The birth of the book was initiated by young dermatologists, eager to start their practice, who always questioned me during various scientific meetings. It incubated and took shape through interactions with all my colleagues, who shared their expertise and knowledge gathered worldwide. I am also indebted to Dr Philippe Deprez for teaching the fine art of combining sand abrasion with chemical peels. All this crystallized with unwavering support from my patients who reposed complete faith in me.

I am thankful to my teachers, particularly Dr Chetan Oberai and late Dr PN Behl who injected me with academic enthusiasm right from the beginning of my career.

I am indebted to the staff at M/s Jaypee Brothers Medical Publishers (P) Ltd, New Delhi, India, who made my work very easy by their technical expertise.

My deepest thanks goes to my family, my spouse Dr JM Khunger and my children, Dr Monica and Dr Arjun, who let me work unhindered in writing the book.

Contents

1

Importance of Chemical Peels

Niti Khunger

- The Power of Peeling
- Downside to Peeling
- Where do Peels Stand Today?
- Why do We Use Chemical Peels?

Introduction

Chemical peeling is a procedure, where a chemical agent of a defined strength is applied to the skin, which causes a controlled destruction of the layers of the skin that is followed by regeneration and remodeling, with improvement of texture and surface abnormalities. The objective of chemical peeling is to cause destruction at the required depth, followed by remodeling without scarring. The concept of skin peeling by chemicals to beautify the skin has been used since time immemorial. Cleopatra used sour milk, containing lactic acid and French women used old wine containing tartaric acid as beauty baths. The modern era of chemical peeling began with MacKee, a dermatologist who used phenol to treat facial scars.[1] Initially, peeling formulas were closely guarded secrets and these procedures attracted interest because of the remarkable results that were achieved. Finally, scientific investigations were undertaken by plastic surgeons and dermatologists like Stegman.[2] The alpha-hydroxy acids were studied by Van Scott and Yu.[3] Since then various agents have been used for chemical peeling with newer agents being added day-to-day.

The Power of Peeling

Chemical peeling has several advantages:

- It is a simple office procedure, and does not require an elaborate OT set-up.
- The procedure is easy to learn and practice, with a short learning curve, particularly for beginners.
- It is safe and effective with minimal complications.
- Superficial peels are noninvasive and can be used as lunchtime procedures.
- No significant postoperative care is required, except for deep peels.
- Except for phenol peels, there is no risk of systemic toxicity.
- Chemical agents are easy to procure and are stable.
- There is a wide array of chemical agents that can be used for peeling, hence treatment can be individualized, according to skin type.
- Unlike lasers, no machines and maintenance is required, hence affordable to every physician.
- Procedure and chemicals are inexpensive and easily affordable to most patients.
- Chemical peeling has been well studied and there is vast long-term experience with peeling agents.
- It can be combined with other modalities such as microneedling, lasers and microdermabrasion.

Downside to Peeling

However, chemical peeling also has few disadvantages:

- Complications such as hyperpigmentation and scarring can occur.

- Except for deep peels, it is a slow process. Multiple sessions are required with superficial peels, to achieve acceptable cosmetic results.
- Results are not permanent and maintenance peels are often required.
- Postpeel, pigmentary changes are common in inexperienced hands, especially in darker skins.
- Skin needs to be primed with medical therapy before peeling and adjunctive therapy is essential to maintain results.
- Deep peels with phenol have a high risk of permanent pigmentary changes in darker skins.

Where do Peels Stand Today?

There has been an explosive interest in procedural techniques for skin rejuvenation and the trend is increasingly for procedures that are noninvasive or minimally invasive, requiring little downtime. The majority of the chemical peeling procedures fit into this category. The long-term experience with chemical peels has shown them to be safe and effective for a variety of common conditions like dyschromias, photoaging and acne.

According to a recent report by the National Ambulatory Medical Care Survey in US, today botulinum toxin injections, chemical peels and fillers are the three most common office based cosmetic procedures being performed.[4]

The advent of nonablative lasers and light therapy systems initially led to a decline in the use of chemical peels. However, as compared to chemical peeling, many of these newer techniques are still in the learning phase and long-term effects are unknown. Newer, safer and more effective peeling agents, such as mandelic acid, lactic acid, phytic acid, pyruvic acid, etc. continue to attract attention of cosmetic dermatologists, the world over. This has led to resurgence in the use of chemical peels.[5] Lasers on the other hand are still very expensive to acquire and maintain. Till these newer nonablative light therapies, become more predictable, affordable and widely available, chemical peels continue to be an extremely useful armamentarium in the treatment of common conditions such as skin rejuvenation, photoaging, melasma and acne.

Why do We Use Chemical Peels?

Chemical peeling is a versatile tool that can help build a good cosmetic practice. Though lasers have caused a large impact, partially fuelled by media hype, chemical peels can still be considered as a simple and effective modality, in any cosmetic physician's repertoire. Often it is not possible for physicians to buy three different lasers to treat each problem. Chemical peels can treat photodamaged skin, pre-skin cancers, acne, melasma and other dyschromias, thus allowing treatment of a number of different problems without any special equipment.[6] New advances in peel approaches, including combination, sequential and segmental peels, safer and lower-strength peeling agents, added to the menu of options, are allowing clinicians to tailor their practices to patients' needs, often without added costs. Chemical peels are thus not only a part of the cosmetic scene of the past, but also a definite cornerstone of the future.

Conclusion

Chemical peeling is a simple and safe office procedure. A thorough knowledge of peeling agents and their mechanisms of action are essential for all physicians practicing cosmetic dermatology. The nuances of peeling, particularly in darker skins, where lasers carry a higher risk of complications, fill a gap in the treatment of common conditions such as facial melanoses, photoaging, acne and skin rejuvenation.

Key Points

√ Chemical peeling is a useful office procedure for the treatment of common conditions such as dyschromias, skin rejuvenation and acne.

√ It has a short learning curve and can be easily practiced, even by beginners.

√ It is safe and effective with minimal complications.

√ Inexpensive and affordable to doctor and patient alike.

References

1. Brody H. History of chemical peels. In: Baxter S (Ed). Chemical peeling and resurfacing. 2nd edn. St. Louis: Mosby Year Book; 1997.pp.1-5.

2. Stegman SJ. A comparative histologic study of the effects of the three peeling agents and dermabrasion on normal and sun damaged skin. Aesth Plast Surg. 1982;6:123.

3. Van Scott EJ, Yu RJ. Hyperkeratinization, corneocyte adhesion and hydroxy acids. J Am Acad Dermatol. 1984;11:867-79.

4. Ahn CSI, Davis SA, Dabade TS, Wiliford PM, Feldman SR. Cosmetic procedures performed in the United States: 16 year analysis. Dermatol Surg. 2013;39:1351-9.

5. Sapijaszko MJA. Chemical peels—a re-emerging art. Skin Care Guide.com

6. Hantash B, Stewart DB, Cooper ZA, et al. Facial resurfacing for nonmelanoma skin cancer prophylaxis. Arch Dermatol. 2006;142: 976-82.

2

Basics of Chemical Peeling

Monica Khunger

- Acids and Bases
- Basic Chemistry of Skin
- Mechanism of Action of Peeling Agents
- Wound Healing

Introduction

The basic principle of chemical peeling is to cause injury to the skin at the required depth, allowing regeneration to take place, without causing permanent scarring. The various types of chemical agents used in chemical peeling vary in their chemical properties and mechanism of action. In order to minimize the tremendous variability of response of the skin to these agents, it is essential to understand basic chemistry of these agents, anatomy of the skin and the skin-chemical interactions.[1]

Acids and Bases[1]

An acid is a chemical capable of releasing a H^+ ion (proton). The pH is a measure of the acidity or alkalinity of a solution. Aqueous solutions at 25° with a pH less than 7 are considered acidic, while those with a pH greater than seven are considered basic or alkaline. The pH of 7 is considered neutral at 25°.

A lower pH causes more irritation, but is more effective. Some formulations add buffers like phosphoric acid to increase the pH and reduce irritation. The pKa of the solution is the pH at which half is in acid form; therefore, a lower pKa means that more free acid is available. Many products advertise the acid percentage; however, pKa is a more accurate determinant of strength.

The pKa or dissociation constant of a substance is its capacity to donate protons. The pKa is the pH at which the level of free acid is same as the level of the salt of the substance.

$$pH = pKa + log\,(salt)/(acid)$$

The pH is equal to the pKa when the concentration of the base is equal to the concentration of the acid in a given solution.

It is important to remember that concentration of the peeling agent can vary between various brands and formulations, even though the label indicates the same concentration. Different methods used to determine concentration of acid can also produce some variation. From strongest to weakest, these methods are dilutions of a saturated solution, weight-to-weight method, weight-to-volume method, and grams of acid crystal mixed to 100 mL of water. Hence, it is essential for the physician to use the same formulation for peeling, the patient on consecutive peels, in order to get consistent results.

Basic Chemistry of Skin[1]

The skin can be considered as an aqueous solution, consisting mainly of dissolved proteins, carbohydrates, lipids and minerals.

APPROXIMATE COMPOSITION OF SKIN

- Water 70%
- Proteins 25.5%
- Lipids 2%

- Carbohydrates 2%
- Minerals and elements (copper, zinc, etc.) 0.5%.

The pH of the epidermis is acidic (approximately 5) due to secretion of sebum and sweat. This acid mantle of the skin protects it from bacteria and fungi. Dry skin is more acidic as compared to oily skin. The pH of the dermis is less acidic as compared to the epidermis, due to higher content of fluid and blood. The pH of the papillary dermis is 6 and reticular dermis is 7.

Mechanism of Action of Peeling Agents[1-4]

Peeling agents act by three mechanisms:
1. Metabolic
2. Caustic
3. Toxic.

METABOLIC ACTION

Alpha Hydroxy Acids

Alpha hydroxy acids (AHA) are also called as fruit acids as they are found in fruits. They are weak acids with a pKa of 3.8. They act by interfering with the functioning of enzymes such as kinases, sulfotransferases and phosphotransferases, which attach sulfate and phosphate molecules to the corneocytes. This causes desquamation of corneocytes, leading to epidermal desiccation and shedding. In higher concentrations of free acid, they act as caustic agents. Alpha hydroxy acids also cause stimulation of epidermal growth and smoothening of the skin. In the dermis, there is an induction of inflammatory response with deposition of glycosaminoglycans and new collagen formation. Through fibroblast modulation, they alter the dermal matrix and collagen. They do not have a self-neutralizing action like trichloroacetic acid and have to be neutralized. This increases the risk of side effects such as inflammation, pigmentary changes and scarring.

Azelaic Acid

Azelaic acid is a saturated dicarboxylic acid, found naturally in wheat rye and barley. The exact mechanism of action is not known, but it has a bactericidal action against *Propionibacterium acnes* and *Staphylococcus epidermidis* and bacteriostatic action against *Staph. aureus, E. coli, Pseudomonas aeruginosa* and *Candida albicans*. It also has antiviral, antiproliferative, and free radical scavenging activity *in vitro*. Hence it is useful in acne and melasma.

Retinoic Acid

Retinoids are diterpenes and vitamin A or retinol is present in food as beta carotene. In the skin it is converted to retinaldehyde and subsequently 95% of this is converted to retinyl ester and 5% to all-transretinoic acid (tretinoin) and 9-cis-retinoic acid. In chemical peeling, retinol and all-transretinoic acid are used in high concentrations. They bind to the retinoic acid receptors (RAR) in the nucleus and have multiple actions.

CAUSTIC ACTION

Trichloroacetic Acid

Trichloroacetic acid (TCA) is a strong acid with pKa 0.26, available as anhydrous white crystals. It has a caustic action and causes coagulation of proteins, seen visually as frosting. It is self-neutralizing and is not absorbed into the systemic circulation.

TOXIC ACTION

Phenol

It has properties of a weak acid, soluble in ethanol, with a high pKa of 9.9. It is also called as carbolic acid when dissolved in water. Phenol has antiseptic, antifungal and anesthetic properties. It acts by enzyme inactivation, protein denaturation and increased permeability of cell membranes leading to cell death. It is absorbed in the systemic circulation and can cause cardiac, renal and hepatic toxicity.

Resorcinol

It has similar actions as phenol, with reduced toxicity.

Salicylic Acid

It is a beta-hydroxy acid with a pKa of 3, soluble in ethanol. It has keratolytic properties and is lipophilic, thus easily penetrating the sebaceous follicles and hence useful in acne. It causes dissolution of the intercellular cement substance and hence reduces corneocyte adhesion. It has comedolytic and anti-inflammatory properties. It is available as a powder, which is dissolved in ethanol to prepare a solution. On application the vehicle evaporates leaving a precipitate of salicylic acid that is seen as white pseudofrost. When applied over large areas, it can be systemically absorbed causing salicylism.

Wound Healing[3,5-7]

Wound healing has basically three phases, after any injury to the skin:
1. Inflammatory phase
2. Proliferative phase
3. Maturational phase.

The stages of wound healing after a chemical peel, depend on the depth of skin necrosis. In superficial and medium depth peels, initially there is coagulation and inflammation, followed by re-epithelialization. Glycolic acid also causes remodeling of the dermis by fibroblast modulation. In deep peels, coagulation and inflammation are followed by granulation tissue formation, angiogenesis and subsequent re-epithelialization along with remodeling of collagen and matrix in the dermis. The three stages of inflammation, tissue proliferation and tissue remodeling are an overlapping series of continuous processes (Figures 2.1A to D).

COAGULATION AND INFLAMMATION

There is coagulation and precipitation of proteins that leads to necrosis and degeneration of the stratum corneum and keratinocytes. Similar process occurs in the dermis in deeper peels. Clotting factors, monophages, lymphocytes, various cytokines and inflammatory mediators are activated. Platelets are the first to respond, releasing multiple chemokines, including epidermal growth factor (EGF), fibronectin, fibrinogen, histamine, platelet-derived growth factor (PDGF), serotonin, etc. Neutrophils act as scavengers and decontaminate the wound. The macrophages secrete numerous enzymes and cytokines, including collagenases, which debride the wound, interleukins and tumor necrosis factor (TNF), stimulating fibroblasts to produce collagen and promote angiogenesis and transforming growth factor (TGF), which stimulates the keratinocytes. This is followed by the proliferative phase.

TISSUE PROLIFERATION

Epithelialization

It occurs early in the wound healing mechanism. In superficial peels, where the basement membrane is intact, epithelial cells migrate upwards and normal epidermis is restored in 2 to 3 days. If the wound is below the basement membrane as in medium and deep peels, re-epithelialization takes place by migration of keratinocytes from surrounding intact skin and appendages.

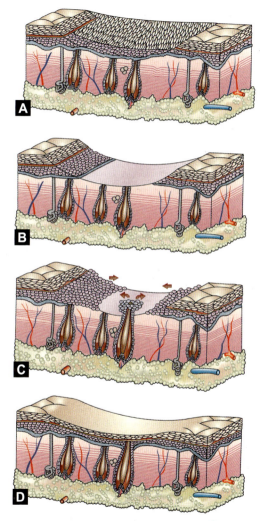

Figs 2.1A to D Histopathology of chemical peels: (A) Skin before chemical peel; (B) Denudation of epidermis and papillary dermis; (C) Epidermal proliferation and migration at 72 hours; (D) Re-epithelialization

Angiogenesis

The process of angiogenesis begins with endothelial cell migration to the wound site and is essential for wound healing. The erythema following a chemical peel primarily is caused by the new capillary growth in the area.

Granulation Tissue

It usually appears on the second day and consists of fibroblasts, which differentiate and produce ground substance and collagen. Growth factors, inflammatory cells, fibronectin, glycosaminoglycans and collagen are all involved in this phase.

TISSUE REMODELING

Collagen remodeling: Collagen remodeling is the main reason that chemical peels are able to cause rejuvenation and reduce wrinkles. The process of remodeling involves a reorientation of the collagen in a parallel fashion and begins as collagen is formed, following the peel. Though collagen remodeling continues, net increase in collagen deposition plateaus after 21 days. However, there are a lot of factors that still need to be elucidated.

Conclusion

In spite of the advances in our understanding of chemical peels, there is still variation in the pH, pKa and concentration of free acid in various solutions. Many times, the use of chemical peels becomes intuitive rather than scientific, which can lead to a higher risk of side effects. Understanding the basic processes of wound healing, following chemical peels, will lead to better interventions to hasten wound repair and restoration of normal skin. The advent of newer, safer, effective standardized peeling agents will go a long way in the scientific use of chemical peeling as an important tool for skin rejuvenation and treatment of pigmentary changes and acne.

> ### Key Points
>
> √ The pKa is the pH at which the level of free acid is the same as the level of the salt of the substance. It is a more accurate determinant of strength.
> √ Peeling agents act by different mechanisms metabolic, caustic and toxic.

References

1. Dewandre L. The chemistry of peels and a hypothesis of action mechanisms. In: Rubin MG (Ed). Chemical Peels. 1st edn. Elsevier Inc; 2006.pp.1-12.
2. Brody HJ. Skin response to chemical peeling. In: Coleman WP, Lawrence N (Eds). Skin Resurfacing. 1st edn. Baltimore: Williams and Wilkins; 1998.pp.37-44.
3. Savant SS. Superficial and medium depth chemical peeling. In: Savant SS (Ed). Textbook of Dermatosurgery and Cosmetology. 2nd edn. ASCAD; 2005.pp.177-95.
4. Baumann L. Chemical peeling. In: Baumann L (Ed). Cosmetic Dermatology. Principles and Practice. 1st edn. New York: The McGraw-Hill Conpanies; 2002.pp.173-86.
5. Cohen IK, Diegelmann RF, Lindblad WJ (Eds). Wound Healing: Biochemical and Clinical Aspects. Philadelphia, PA: WB Saunders, 1992.
6. Brody H. Wound healing. Chemical Peeling and Resurfacing. 2nd edn. St. Louis: Mosby Year Book Inc; 1997.pp.29-38.
7. Stegman S. A comparative histologic study of the effects of three peeling agents and dermabrasion on normal and sun damaged skin. Aesth Plast Surg. 1982;6:123.

3

Types of Peels

Niti Khunger

- Peeling Agents
- Histological Classification of Peels
- Factors Modifying Depth of Peels
- Facial and Nonfacial Peels
- Regional Peels
- Combination Peels
- Sequential Peels
- Segmental Peels
- Switch Peels

Introduction

Chemical peels are classified according to the histological level of the necrosis of the skin.[1] There are two classifications; Brody's classification[2] differs slightly from Rubin's classification.[1] The peeling agent is the most important factor in determining the depth of the peel, but other variables such as skin type, prepeel priming and method of application also play a role. Superficial and medium depth peels are safer for Indian skins. In darker skins deep peels should be avoided, as they are associated with a high-risk of complications.

Peeling Agents

There is a wide array of peeling agents available in the market today, with different formulations and combinations. It is essential for the physician to be familiar with the peeling agents they use as there can be tremendous variability between formulations and brands, that can lead to unexpected outcomes and complications. Some common peeling agents are:

- Alpha hydroxy acid (AHA, also called as fruit acids as they are found in certain fruits) glycolic acid 35 to 70%, lactic acid 10 to 90%, mandelic acid 30 to 50%, tartaric acid, malic acid, phytic acid
- Beta hydroxy acids—salicylic acid 20 to 50%, citric acid 20 to 70%
- Trichloroacetic acid (TCA) 10 to 35%
- Alpha ketoacids—pyruvic acid 40 to 70%
- Jessner's solution (lactic acid 14 gm, salicylic acid 14 gm, resorcinol 14 gm)
- Modified Jessner's solutions
- Retinoic acid 1 to 5%, retinol
- Resorcinol is replaced with citric acid 8%
- Phenol 88%
- Combinaton peels.

Histological Classification of Peels[1] (Table 3.1)

Very superficial peels cause exfoliation of the stratum corneum, without any epidermal necrosis. This is followed by epidermal thickening and qualitative regenerative changes. Superficial chemical peels cause destruction of the full epidermis, up to the basal layer. Destruction of the epidermis, papillary dermis up to the upper one-third of the reticular dermis constitutes a medium depth peel. Necrosis of the entire epidermis and papillary dermis, with inflammation extending to the mid-reticular dermis causes a deep peel (Figure 3.1).

Table 3.1: Histological classification of peels

Types of peel	Histological level	Agents
Very superficial	Exfoliation of the stratum corneum, without any epidermal necrosis	Glycolic acid 30–50% applied for 1–2 minutes TCA 10% applied as 1 coat Jessner's solution 1–3 coats Resorcinol 20–30% applied for 5–10 minutes
Superficial	Necrosis of part or entire epidermis, not below the basal layer	Glycolic acid 50–70% applied for 2–10 minutes, depending on the type and thickness of the skin TCA 10–30% Jessner's solution 4–10 coats Resorcinol 40–50% applied for 30–60 minutes
Medium	Necrosis of the epidermis, papillary dermis up to the upper reticular dermis	Glycolic acid 70% applied for 3–30 minutes, depending on the type and thickness of the skin TCA 35–50% Glycolic acid 70% plus TCA 35% Jessner's solution plus TCA 35% CO_2 plus TCA 35%
Deep	Necrosis of the epidermis, papilary dermis up to mid-reticular dermis	Phenol 88% Baker Gordon phenol formula

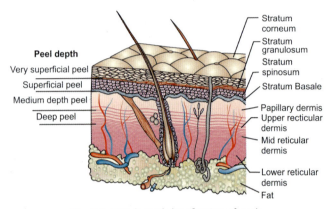

Fig. 3.1 Histological classification of peels

Factors Modifying Depth of Peels

The depth of a peel depends on many factors:[3,4]

PEELING AGENT

The peeling agent and its concentration is the most important factor in determining the peel depth. The higher the concentration, greater is the depth. However, peeling agents can be combined at lower concentrations, to achieve greater depths, reducing side effects associated with higher concentrations.

It should be kept in mind that concentration of the peeling agent can vary, with different brands and formulations of the same peeling agent. This is because different methods used to determine concentration of acid can produce some variation. Hence, while peeling a patient, one must not interchange the brand of the peeling agent, even if it indicates the same concentration. This can lead to an inadvertent variation in concentration, with potential increased risk of complications.

AVAILABILITY OF FREE ACID

The pKa of the solution is the pH at which half is in acid form. Hence, a lower pKa means that more free acid is available for action. Though many products advertise the acid percentage, the pKa is a more accurate determinant of strength of the peeling agent.

DURATION OF CONTACT

For AHA peels such as glycolic acid, prolonging the duration of contact increases the depth of the peel. Hence, timing of the peel is as important as the concentration. This is not required for agents such as TCA and salicylic acid, where concentration is important.

TECHNIQUE OF APPLICATION

If the peel is rubbed into the skin, it achieves a greater depth, than if it is painted on the skin. The number of coats applied and degree of frosting, as in Jessner's solution and salicyclic acid peel can be varied, increasing the peel depth.

METHOD OF PRIMING THE PATIENT

The application of low concentrations of glycolic acid, tretinoin or salicylic acid during the period of prepeel priming thins the stratum corneum, causing a uniform, even and greater penetration of the chemical agent.

METHOD OF DEGREASING THE SKIN

Vigorous degreasing of the skin can increase penetration and cause 'hotspots' to develop.

CHARACTERISTICS OF PATIENT'S SKIN

In thick oily skin, penetration is less as compared to thin dry skin. The level of photodamage, actinic damage and presence of irregular superficial lesions such as seborrheic keratoses, dermatoses papulosa nigra, lentigo, etc. cause irregular penetration of peeling agent.

LOCATION OF PEEL

A facial peel will show greater depth as compared to a nonfacial peel, where the skin is thicker.

Hence, it is essential to standardize the peeling agents, procedure of priming the patient, cleaning and degreasing the skin so as to maintain the required depth of the peel.

Facial and Nonfacial Peels

Following a chemical peel, the epidermis re-epithelializes from the pilosebaceous unit, which are maximum on the face (Figures 3.2A and B). Hence healing on the nonfacial areas is delayed as compared to the facial areas. The delayed healing on the nonfacial areas, leads to a higher risk of complications, like infection, pigmentary changes and keloid formation. Dermal peels are particularly prone to scarring and textural changes, hence deep peels should be avoided in nonfacial areas. Photodamaged skin in nonfacial areas like the neck, décolleté area of the chest, upper back and exposed areas of the forearms is improved more safely with repeated superficial peels, rather than deeper peels. These nonfacial areas are larger than the face, hence absorption and toxicity with agents like salicylic acid and resorcinol is more likely, when applied to larger areas.

Regional Peels

Regional peels or spot peels are applied to localized areas. Superficial and medium peels can be safely applied, however,

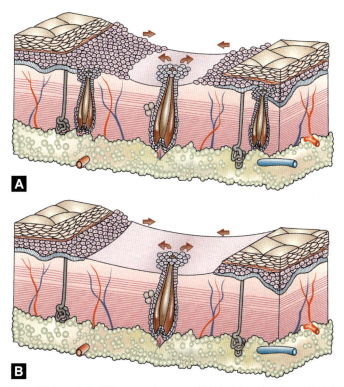

Figs 3.2A and B Difference between (A) facial and (B) nonfacial skin. Facial skin has a greater density of pilosebaceous units, hence epithelialization occurs earlier as compared to nonfacial skin

deep peels should be avoided on cosmetically important areas as they may cause permanent pigmentary alterations. Lines of demarcation are common with localized peels, particularly in dark skin individuals. Hence feathering should be done at the edges and bleaching agents should be applied at the borders.

Combination Peels

Combination peels combine two or more different agents in a single formulation. The advantages of combination peels are multiple. The range of action of a single peel can be increased by combining agents that complement their actions. The depth and efficacy of the peel can be increased. It can also improve the safety of formulations as lower concentrations of individual agents are used. The earliest and most widely used combination peel is Jessner's solution. However, many of these combination peels are proprietary. They contain lower concentrations and are left over peels that can be safely used in darker skin types. Some peels are in gel formulations where the chemical agents are slowly released reducing side effects.

Sequential Peels

Sequential peels are chemical peels using more than one peel at a time in a sequential manner as they may not be compatible in a single formulation. The need for the sequential peel arises from the fact that the pKa of different chemicals may not be similar hence the use of optimal strength of these chemicals in a single formulation may not practicable. The advantage is that the peel that is applied first exfoliates the skin and enhances penetration of the second peel leading to a greater depth of the peel. These are medium depth peels and should be used with proper precautions and priming in dark skin patients. Priming with sunscreens and hypopigmenting agents should be done at least 2 to 4 weeks prior to sequential peels.

Segmental Peels

Segmental peels consist of using different peels in different cosmetic units, at the same session. The choice of the peeling agent depends on the condition being treated, the severity in different cosmetic units and the type of patient's skin, e.g. a patient with melasma and acne can be treated with a peel containing glycolic acid, hydroquinone and kojic acid on the cheek and comedones on the nose and forehead are treated with salicylic acid 20 to 30%.

Switch Peels

The beauty of chemical peeling is that it is easily possible to switch from one peel to the other, tailoring the peeling agents according to the requirement of the patient, as the condition improves. When the peels are changed serially in different peeling sessions, they are called switch peels. It gives a greater flexibility in choosing a peeling protocol from patient to patient, hence leading to greater patient and professional satisfaction.

Conclusion

Peels are classified according to the histological depth of necrosis achieved by the peeling agent. There is a plethora of peeling agents that are available in varying concentrations. The peeling agent and its concentration must be selected according to the pathology being treated. The depth of the peel can be varied by many factors, the most important being the peeling agent and its concentration. The brand or method of preparing the peeling agent should not be interchanged while peeling a patient, as the amount of free acid can differ even if the label indicates the same concentration. It is important for the physician to be familiar with a few standardized brands and also standardize the method of priming the skin and technique of application of peeling agent so as to maintain the required depth of peel.

Key Points

√ Classification of peels depends on histological depth of necrosis, very superficial, superficial, medium and deep.
√ The peeling agent and its concentration are the most important factors for determining depth of the peel.
√ All efforts should be made to standardize the peeling agent, method of priming and technique of application.
√ Glycolic acid, TCA and salicylic acid peels are the most commonly used peeling agents.

References

1. Rubin MG. Glycolic acid peels. In: Winter SR, James M, Caputo GR (Eds). Manual of Chemical Peels—Superfical and Medium Depth, 1st edn. Philadelphia: JB Lippincot Co; 1995.pp.89-102.
2. Brody H. Histology and classification. In: Baxter S (Ed). Chemical Peeling and Resurfacing. 2nd edn, St. Louis: Mosby Year Book Inc; 1997. pp.7-27.
3. Savant SS. Superficial and medium depth chemical peeling. In: Savant SS (Ed). Textbook of Dermatosurgery and Cosmetology, 2nd edn. ASCAD; 2005.pp.177-95.
4. Baumann L. Chemical peeling. In: Baumann L (Ed). Cosmetic Dermatology. Principles and Practice, 1st edn. New York: The McGraw-Hill Companies; 2002.pp.173-86.

4

Choosing the Right Peeling Agent

Niti Khunger

- Indications
- Contraindications
- Patient Assessment
- Counseling
- Skin Types
- Expected Outcomes in Chemical Peeling

Introduction

Chemical peeling is a useful technique in the treatment of common cosmetic disorders such as melasma, photodamage, acne, mild facial scarring and skin rejuvenation. Various peeling agents acting at different depths can be utilized. Some peels may be more appropriate for certain conditions and for particular skin types. Hence, the choice of peeling agent has to be individualized and a patient may require different peeling agents over a period of time for maximum benefit. Thus, it is important to choose the right peel for the right patient.

Indications[1-4]

1. *Pigmentary disorders:*
    - Resistant melasma (Figure 4.1)
    - Pigmented cosmetic dermatitis

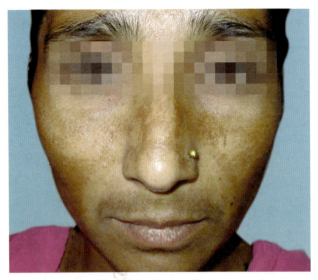

Fig. 4.1 Resistant melasma

- Freckles
- Lentigines
- Postinflammatory hyperpigmentation

2. *Acne:*
   - Comedonal acne
   - Macular hyperpigmented postacne scars (Figures 4.2A and B)
   - Superficial mild postacne scarring
   - Icepick scars
   - Acne excoriée
   - Acne cosmetica

3. *Cosmetic:*
   - Photoaging (Figure 4.3)
   - Fine wrinkling
   - Moderate actinic damage
   - Actinic keratoses

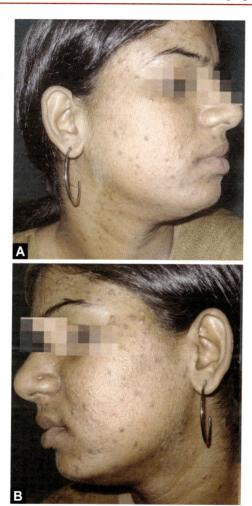

Figs 4.2A and B Pigmented acne scars

- Skin glow
- Oily skin
- Rough skin

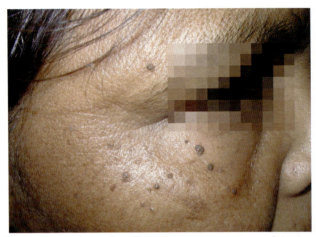

Fig. 4.3 Photoaging with senile lentigines, dermatosis papulosa nigra, fine wrinkles and early melasma in darker skins

4.   Miscellaneous
   • Keratosis pilaris
   • Macular amyloidosis
   • Ichthyosis
   • Seborrheic keratoses
   • Dilated pores.

Superficial chemical peels are often referred to as lunch-time peels, because they require virtually no downtime. They are useful in the treatment of pigmentary disorders like melasma, where lasers have a high-risk of postinflammatory hyperpigmentation (PIH), particularly in dark-skinned patients. In conditions where there is pigmentary incontinence and increased dermal melanin, they cause inflammation, leading to increased phagocytosis of melanin by macrophages and thus hasten improvement.

In acne, they act as excellent adjuvant techniques for the treatment of comedonal acne. They play an important role in the treatment of mild superficial acne scarring and bring about gradual improvement over a period of time without disturbing the routine of the patient. However, care has to be taken in inflammatory acne, where it can lead to aggravation of inflammation. In acne excoriée, pigmentation is a major component and chemical peels are useful adjuncts in resistant cases.

Chemical peels are the cornerstone of skin rejuvenation programs and produce good results for early signs of aging. Younger patients in their 20s and 30s with fine lines or uneven skin pigmentation caused by sun damage are ideal candidates for these procedures. For moderate wrinkles, deep peels are advocated, however, they are used with extreme caution in type IV–V skins.

Contraindications

- Active bacterial infection, such as folliculitis
- Active herpes simplex (Figure 4.4)

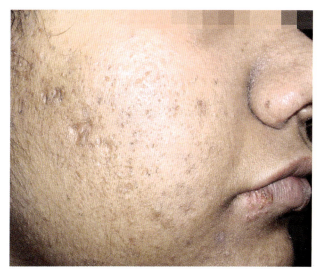

Fig. 4.4 Herpes simplex in a patient scheduled for chemical peel

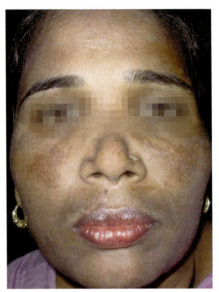

Fig. 4.5 Contraindication to chemical peeling, patient on oral contraceptives

- Viral warts or molluscum contagiosum on the area to be peeled
- Open wounds
- History of taking photosensitive drugs and oral contraceptives (Figure 4.5)
- Uncooperative patient, e.g. patient is careless about sun exposure or application of medicine as directed
- Patient with unrealistic expectations
- For medium depth and deep peels, history of abnormal scarring, atrophic skin and isotretinoin use in the last six months.[5]

Patient Assessment[6] (Table 4.1)

While evaluating a patient, an extensive history should be taken at the first visit. It is easier to fill a proforma so that no issues

Table 4.1: Assessment of patient

History

1. *Level of sun exposure:*	Maximum (>3 hours/day)
	Moderate (1–3 hours/day)
	Minimal (<1 hour/day)
	Yes/No
2. History of oral herpes simplex frequency of episodes	Yes/No
3. Recent isotretinoin treatment in the last 6 months (in patients planned for medium depth and deep peels)	Yes/No
4. Keloidal tendency	Yes/No
5. Tendency for postinflammatory hyperpigmentation	Yes/No
6. Current medications	Yes/No
7. Previous surgical treatment	Yes/No
8. Immunocompromising conditions	Yes/No
9. Smoking	Yes/No

Examination

1. Skin type I/II/III/IV/V/VI
2. Degree of photoaging, Level 1/2/3/4/5/6
3. Sebaceous activity oily/dry/normal skin
4. Previous scars PIH/keloids
5. Infection
6. Pre-existing inflammation

Investigation

1. Skin biopsy when indicated, to confirm diagnoses and see level of pigmentation
2. No specific investigations are indicated for superficial peels; In patients in whom deep peels are planned, routine investigations including hemogram, urinalysis, liver and renal function tests, ECG should be carried out.

are missed. A history of herpes simplex is important as these patients should be given prophylactic acyclovir or valacyclovir to prevent an outbreak of herpes, which can lead to scarring. However, in my opinion, this is necessary only for deeper peels where there is a breach of epidermis and may not be necessary in very light superficial peels. Conditions that cause delayed healing such as chronic smoking, and radiation over the area to be peeled should be ruled out. Immunocompromised states like HIV infection, delay wound healing and increase risk of wound infection. Hence such patients are at a high-risk of complications during deeper peels. Patients on photosensitizing drugs or suffering from photosensitive disorders are at higher risk of PIH, particularly in darker skin types. Contraindication of chemical peeling in patients using isotretinoin is controversial. Though there have been reports of abnormal scarring in patients on isotretinoin, following resurfacing procedures, practically, it is hardly seen with chemical peels. Precautions may be required when performing deep phenol peels. Similarly, patients who have undergone recent facelift or any surgery where extensive undermining of the face that compromises blood supply and delays wound healing has been done should avoid deep chemical peels for at least 6 to 12 months.

IMAGING TECHNIQUES FOR CHEMICAL PEELS

Objective imaging techniques can be extremely useful in assessing the treatment response to chemical peels. Though standardized photography is the mainstay in assessing treatment response, it may not always be objective. The Canfield Reveal® Imager with its software is a very useful tool as it gives standardized photographs in the normal, polarized, melanin and vascular mode. The dermoscope in the polarizing mode can be another useful technique as it gives subsurface features. Recently, the *in vivo* reflectance confocal microscope has been utilized to assess response to chemical peels. Pigmented keratinocytes and melanocytes appear as bright white structures relative to the surrounding skin and a reduction in pigment results in a decreased quantity and intensity of bright white structures and appear more similar to the surrounding normal skin.[6]

Counseling

Counseling the patient is very important prior to chemical peeling. The patient should be psychologically evaluated to judge the motivation and expectations of the patient. A media-hyped patient with unrealistic expectations invariably leads to dissatisfaction. It is advisable to downplay the degree of improvement expected. Discussions about the nature of treatment, expected outcome, time taken for recovery of normal skin, likely complications, pigmentary changes and importance of maintenance regimens are essential. It is essential to have an expectation alignment between the patient and the physician. If the patient is not convinced, it is better to schedule another counseling session. The help of a professional counselor may be sought in case of problematic patients.

Skin Types

Apart from a general physical examination, the skin type of the patient should be evaluated (Table 4.2, Figure 4.6).

The Fitzpatrick skin phototype classification will give an idea about the amount of tanning of the patient, expected response to the peel, and likely complications. Very superficial and superficial peels are safe in all skin types. All depths of peels can be safely done in patients with skin type I–II, patients with skin type III–IV, may show heightened response with medium and deeper peels, particularly on sun exposure. Medium peels should be done with extreme caution in skin types V–VI and

Table 4.2: Fitzpatrick skin phototypes

Skin type	Reaction to sun exposure	Description
I	Always burns, never tans	Very white and freckled
II	Always burns, minimally tans	White
III	Moderately burns, uniformly tans	Light brown
IV	Minimally burns, always tans	Moderate brown
V	Rarely burns, profusely tans	Dark brown
VI	Never burns, deeply pigmented	Black skin

Skin Type		Heritage
1		Celtic, Scandinavian and infants
2		Northern European
3		Central European
4		Mediterranean, Asian
5		South American, Indian, Native American
6		African, Afro-American, Aborigine

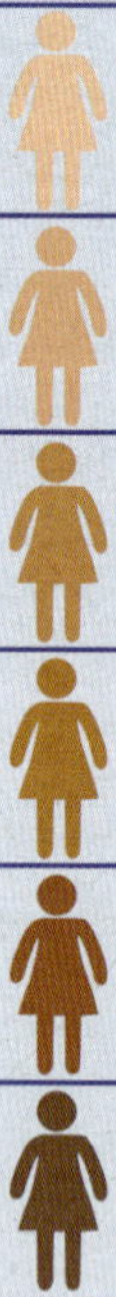

Fig. 4.6 Skin phototypes

deep peels are better avoided, due to high-risk of permanent pigmentary changes.

The level of photodamage will help in selecting the proper depth of the peel required for optimum improvement (Table 4.3, Figures 4.7 to 4.10).

Table 4.3: Glogau photoaging classification
I   *Mild (Age 28–35 years):* • Little wrinkling, no scarring • No keratoses • Requires little or no make-up
II   *Moderate (Age 35–50 years):* • Early wrinkling, minimal scarring • Shallow color with early actinic keratoses • Little make-up
III   *Advanced (Age 50–60 years):* • Persistent wrinkling at rest, moderate acne scarring • Discoloration with telangiectasia and actinic keratoses • Always wears make-up
IV   *Severe (Age 60–75 years):* • Dynamic and gravitational wrinkling, severe acne scarring • Multiple actinic keratoses • Wears make-up with poor coverage

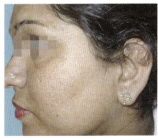

Fig 4.7 Levels of photoaging Grade 1

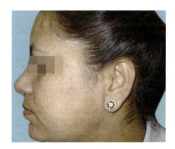

Fig 4.8 Levels of photoaging Grade 2

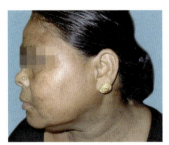

Fig 4.9 Levels of photoaging
Grade 3

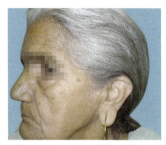

Fig 4.10 Levels of photoaging
Grade 4

Expected Outcomes in Chemical Peeling

When initiating chemical peels in a cosmetic practice, the beginner is often confused about the selection of the peeling agent and its strength. The most important factor is the pathology of the treating condition, which also determines the expected outcome of the peeling procedures (Table 4.4).

EPIDERMAL PEELS

Excellent Results

- Epidermal melasma
- Ephelides
- Dull uneven complexion
- Epidermal hyperpigmentation
- Comedonal acne.

Variable Results

- Senile lentigines
- Mixed melasma (epidermal and dermal)
- Postinflammatory hyperpigmentation

Poor Results

- Dermal melasma
- Dermal pigmentation
- Seborrheic keratosis
- Nevi.

MEDIUM PEELS

Excellent Results

- Epidermal melasma
- Ephelides
- Senile lentigines
- Epidermal hyperpigmentation
- Postacne pigmentation
- Superficial scars
- Mild wrinkles.

Variable Results

- Seborrheic keratosis
- Mixed melasma (epidermal and dermal)
- Postinflammatory hyperpigmentation
- Acne scars.

Poor Results

- Nevi
- Deep wrinkles
- Deep and icepick acne scars.

Conclusion

The re-emergence of chemical peeling in cosmetic practice has mainly occurred due to well-documented scientific studies of the outcomes of chemical peeling in dyschromias

Contd...

Table 4.4: Ready-reckoner for selection of peeling agent

Condition	Depth	Peeling depth required	Peeling agent	Result	Prognosis
Freckles	Up to basal layer	Superficial	GA 50–70% TCA 10–30% SA 30–50%	Good	Recurrence at other sites
Lentigo	Up to papillary dermis	Superficial to medium	GA 70% TCA 35–50% Jessner's + TCA 35%	Good	Recurrence at other sites
Melasma epidermal	Up to basal layer	Superficial	GA 50–70% TCA 10–30% SA 30–50% MA 40%	Good	Recurrence likely
Melasma dermal/mixed	Up to mid-dermis	Medium-deep	GA 50–70% TCA 10–30% SA 30–50% combinations	Partial-poor	Recurrence common
PIH	Variable	Superficial to medium	GA 50–70% TCA 10–30% SA 30–50%	Variable	Good

Contd...

Contd...

Condition	Depth	Peeling depth required	Peeling agent	Result	Prognosis
Acne comedonal	Stratum corneum	Very superficial	SA 20–30% GA 30–50% applied for 1–2 minutes TCA 10%	Good	Good
Acne active	Up to basal layer	Superficial	MA 40% SA 30–50% GA 50–70% TCA 10–30%	Good	Good
Acne scars superficial	Up to papillary dermis	Superficial to medium	GA 70% TCA 35–50% Jessner's + TCA 35% combinations	Good	Good
Skin rejuvenation	Up to basal layer	Superficial	GA 50–70% TCA 10–30% SA 30–50%	Good	Good

Contd...

Condition	Depth	Peeling depth required	Peeling agent	Result	Prognosis
Wrinkles mild	Up to basal layer	Superficial	GA 50–70% TCA 10–30% SA 30–50%	Good	Good
Wrinkles moderate	Up to mid-dermis	Medium-deep	GA 50–70% TCA 10–30% SA 30–50% combinations	Partial	Recurrence with age

Abbreviations: GA—Glycolic acid, TCA—Trichloroacetic acid, SA—Salicylic acid, MA—Mandelic acid and superficial scars. However, prior evaluation of the patient, the depth of peeling required, selection of peeling agent and adequate counseling are important prerequisites of successful results. All factors including skin type, level of damage, pathology of the condition to be treated, psychology of the patient, occupation and level of sun exposure and availability of down-time help in selecting the right peel for the right patient.

Key Points

√ Chemical peels are mainly indicated for the treatment of superficial hyperpigmentation, skin rejuvenation and acne.
√ The patient must be evaluated before peeling in order to select the right peel for the right patient.

References

1. Savant SS. Superficial and medium depth chemical peeling. In: Savant SS (Ed). Textbook of Dermatosurgery and Cosmetology, 2nd edn. ASCAD. 2005.pp.177-95.
2. Baumann L. Chemical peeling. In: Baumann L (Ed). Cosmetic Dermatology: Principles and Practice, 1st edn. New York: The McGraw-Hill Companies; 2002.pp.173-86.
3. Brody H. General peeling concepts: Chemical peeling and resurfacing, 2nd edn. St. Louis: Mosby Year Book Inc., 1997.pp.39-72.
4. Roenigk RK. Retinoids, dermabrasion, chemical peel and keloids. In: Roenigk RK, Roenigk HH Jr (Eds). Surgical Dermatology: Advances in Current Practice. St Louis: Mosby, 1993.pp.376-83.
5. Rubin MG. Photoaged and photodamaged skin. In: Mark J Rubin (Ed). Manual of chemical peels-superfical and medium depth, 1st edn. Philadelphia. JB Lippincot Co. 1995.pp.1-16.
6. Goberdhan LT, Mehta RC, Aguilar C, Makino ET, Colvan L. Assessment of a superficial chemical peel combined with a multimodal, hydroquinone-free skin brightener using *in vivo* reflectance confocal microscopy. J Drugs Dermatol. 2013;12(3):S38-41.

5

Getting Started

Niti Khunger

- Equipment and Reagents
- Consent Form
- Documentation and Photographs
- Patient Handouts and Instructions
- Checklist
- Basic Procedure

Introduction

Chemical peeling is a simple dermatosurgical office procedure that is based on scientific studies of wound healing, following application of exfoliating chemical agents to the skin. The basic principle is to cause controlled injury to the skin, which is followed by resurfacing of the epidermis and remodeling of the collagen. The simplicity of chemical peeling is that it hardly requires any instrumentation, and hence can be performed as an office outpatient procedure.

Equipment and Reagents (Figure 5.1)

BASIC FACILITY

- Clinic or outpatient day care facility
- Surgical OT is needed only for performing deep phenol peels.

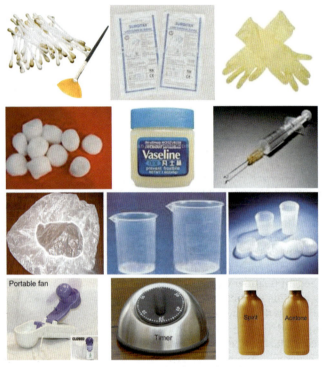

Fig. 5.1 Equipment for chemical peeling

REAGENTS

- Chemical peeling agents with varying concentrations, correctly labeled
- Neutralizing solutions
- Cold water
- Syringe filled with normal saline to irrigate the eyes, if there is accidental spillage of reagent in the eyes.
- Alcohol or spirit for cleansing
- Acetone for degreasing.

EQUIPMENT

- Gloves
- Cap or headband to pull back the patient's hair
- Glass cup to hold the peeling agent
- Cotton tip applicators, ear buds or fine toothpicks
- $2'' \times 2''$ gauze pieces
- Timer for glycolic acid peels
- Hand held fan for patient comfort.

Consent Form (Appendix III)

Informed consent is a legal condition whereby a person gives consent to perform a procedure based upon an understanding of the facts, implications and likely complications arising from the procedure. The individual needs to be in possession of relevant facts and also of his reasoning faculties at the time of signing the consent form. The patient should be explained the need for treatment, consequences of nontreatment and modes of possible treatment. The duration of the procedure, number of sittings that may be required, approximate cost of treatment, expected results, side effects and importance of following instructions before and after the procedure should be clearly discussed. Signing the consent form should not be a routine affair like getting signature on a dotted line by a staff member. Consent form should be signed by the patient and in the case of teenagers (13–18 years), it is better to take the signatures of both the minor and the parent. The patient should feel free to ask questions and emphasis should be on expectation alignment between the patient and physician.

Documentation and Photographs[1,2] (Figures 5.2A to C)

Photographs are very important since patients often do not remember the initial condition. Three views should be taken.

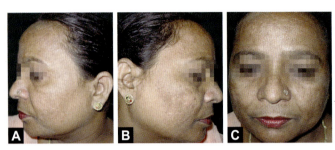

Figs 5.2A to C Standard photographs

Front, right and left side. Every effort should be made to standardize the photographs, including distance, lighting and background. The Canfield imaging system Reveal® is useful to take standardized pictures and also to see for melanin level (Figure 5.3). Photographs should be taken in subsequent treatments also to monitor the progress. It is important to take consent for photographs, which should be incorporated in the consent form. Proper records of the procedure, peeling agent used, concentration, details of treatment given prepeel and postpeel should be maintained. Occurrence of any complications and their treatment should also be recorded.

Patient Handouts and Instructions (Appendix IV)

It is easier to give the patient written instructions, including care of the skin before, during and after a peel.[3] This ensures proper treatment, prevents confusion and also protects the physician, in case patient has not followed instructions properly.

CHOICE OF SUNSCREEN

In a dark skin patient, a sunscreen with sun protection factor 15 (SPF 15) is sufficient. In patients with prolonged exposure to the sun, tendency to postinflammatory hyperpigmentation (PIH) or who tan easily, a higher SPF sunscreen, applied frequently and in adequate quantities is required. In patients with sensitive skins, use a physical sunscreen containing zinc oxide or titanium dioxide only. Patients with oily skins, require a gel based sunscreen, whereas patients with dry skin need a sunscreen with a moisturizing base. If there is excessive peeling, a moisturizing sunscreen is better tolerated as compared to a normal sunscreen.

CHOICE OF CLEANSER

Cleanser should be mild and nonirritating. Scrubs should be strictly avoided. Gentle non-soap cleansers that are less drying are preferred in the peeling phase.

CHOICE OF MOISTURIZER

In patients prone to acne, moisturizers should be nongreasy, whereas in dry skins heavy moisturizers are more suitable.

CHOICE OF RETINOID

In thick oily skins, tretinoin or tazarotene in gel base are preferred, whereas thin dry skins tolerate a cream base. In sensitive skins, retinoids are better avoided or adapalene may be used for short periods. All retinoids should be applied for short duration initially, gradually building up tolerance. They should be stopped at least 1 week before a peel, and restarted only after the skin becomes normal after a peel. Peeling should be postponed if retinoid dermatitis develops. Mild topical steroid like hydrocortisone or fluticasone should be applied and peeling procedure done only after skin normalizes.

CHOICE OF HYPOPIGMENTING AGENT

Hydroquinone is the gold standard and used in a concentration of 5% in patients prone to PIH and dark skin patients. Lower concentration of 2% can be used in patients with sensitive skins. However, some patients are unable to tolerate hydroquinone and develop either irritant or allergic contact dermatitis. In such patients, alternative agents such as kojic acid 1 to 2%, azelaic acid 10 to 20% or arbutin may be used. Low strength glycolic acid 6 to 10% is a useful adjunct.

Checklist

- Is the patient motivated and counseled adequately to come repeatedly for chemical peels and follow instructions?
- Is there a history of herpes?
- Is the patient intolerant/allergic to any topical or systemic drug?
- Any contraindications to peeling?
- Consent form signed?
- Photographs taken?
- Priming done?
- Peeling agent of correct strength selected?
- Neutralizing agents ready?
- Eye irrigation syringe with normal saline ready?
- All precautions taken?
- Postpeel instructions given?

Basic Procedure (Figures 5.3 to 5.5)

Chemical peeling should be undertaken only after the patient has been adequately counseled and primed. The patient signs a consent form and photographs are taken. Contact lenses should be removed before the peel. The patient is asked to wash the face with soap and water, to remove makeup, dirt and grime. The hair is pulled back with a hairband or cap.

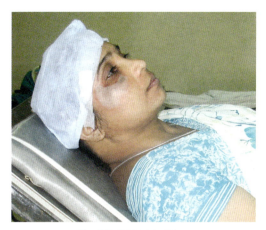

Fig. 5.3 Patient position

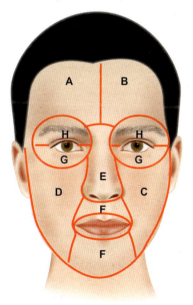

Fig. 5.4 Cosmetic units of the face. Order of application A to H

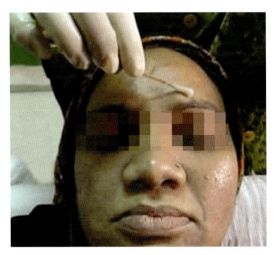

Fig. 5.5 Applying the peel

The patient lies down with head elevated to 45° and eyes closed. First the skin is inspected to see that there are no abrasions or inflammation. Sensitive areas like the inner canthus of the eye and nasolabial folds are protected with petrolatum or vaseline. Using 2″ × 2″ gauze pieces, the skin is cleaned with alcohol and then degreased with acetone. The peeling agent of required strength is poured in a glass beaker and neutralizing agent is also kept ready. Check the label carefully. The peeling agent is then applied either with a brush or cotton tipped applicator or gauze piece. There should be no dripping of the agent. The chemical is applied quickly on the entire face as cosmetic units (*see* Figure 5.4). Begin from the forehead in an upward direction, then the right cheek, nose, left cheek and chin in that order. The perioral, upper and lower eyelids, if required, are treated last. Feathering strokes are applied at the edges, to blend with surrounding skin and prevent demarcation lines. A cooling fan helps to reduce burning of the skin. Do not leave the room and watch out for redness, hot spots and epidermolysis. The peel is neutralized as required according to the peeling agent. The skin is gently dried with gauze and the patient is asked to wash with cold water till the burning subsides. The patient then applies a sunscreen, before leaving the clinic.

Conclusion

Chemical peeling is a simple office procedure that can show gratifying results, without significant downtime. A physician experienced in dealing with all skin types and confident of handling adverse events, as well as an informed, motivated patient with realistic expectations are important to get cosmetically satisfying outcomes.

Key Points

√ Chemical peeling is a simple office procedure.
√ Informed consent, documentation and photographs are important prerequisites to a risk free peel.
√ Physician should be experienced in recognizing clinical condition and depth of peel required, anticipate and treat complications if they arise.

References

1. Scheinfeld N. Photographic images, digital imaging, dermatology, and the law. Arch Dermatol. 2004;140(4):473-6. Review.
2. Niamtu J. Image is everything: Pearls and pitfalls of digital photography and Power Point presentations for the cosmetic surgeon. Dermatol Surg. 2004;30(1):81-91.
3. Rubin MG. Patient information. Manual of chemical peels-superfical and medium depth. Mark J Rubin, Ist edn. Philadelphia. JB Lippincot Co. 1995.pp.60-78.

6

Priming and Skin Preparation

Niti Khunger

- Importance of Priming
- Priming Agents
- Priming Regimen
- Skin Preparation

Introduction

Priming is preparing the skin before starting chemical peels. It is the first step towards performing safe and effective peels. There are two phases to skin priming:

1. Pretreatment, which is application of topical agents, started at least 2 to 4 weeks before the procedure. The goal of this treatment is to assist in producing uniform penetration of the peeling agent, accelerate wound healing and reduce risk of complications.
2. Skin preparation is the steps taken just before applying the peeling agent. The goal of this treatment is cleaning and degreasing the skin in order to enhance penetration of the peeling agent and cause a uniform peel.

Importance of Priming[1-3]

Priming plays a major role in the ultimate results of peeling. There are many advantages to priming the skin.

- *Facilitates uniform penetration of peeling agent:* Retinoic acid or alpha-hydroxy acids like glycolic acid cause thinning of the stratum corneum. When used as priming agents, they help to achieve better and uniform penetration of the peeling agent.

- *Reduces wound healing time:* Retinoic acid applied for at least two weeks prior to peeling has been reported to reduce re-epithelialization time after peeling.[4]

- *Detects intolerance:* Any agent that is likely to be used immediately post-peel or for maintenance therapy, should be applied before the peel. This helps to detect intolerance and is especially important with regard to sunscreen use and hydroquinone (Figures 6.1A and B).

- *Decreases risk of side effects and complications:* The use of hypopigmenting agents like hydroquinone, kojic acid, etc. before the peel greatly reduces the chances of post-inflammatory hyperpigmentation (PIH). This is essential, especially in dark-skinned patients, who have a greater risk of post-inflammatory hyperpigmentation.[5] Hydroquinone, kojic acid, and azelaic acid inhibit tyrosinase and therefore

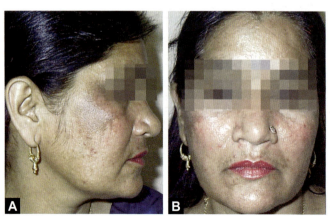

Figs 6.1A and B Intolerance to hydroquinone detected prepeel

reduce melanin formation and hence, substantially decrease the risk of post-inflammatory hyperpigmentation. Retinoic acid and glycolic acid enhance dispersion of melanin granules in the epidermis and are contributory.

- *Enforces patient compliance:* Uncooperative patients who do not follow instructions and observe rules of maintenance therapy are at risk for poor results postpeel and should not be taken up for chemical peeling.

Priming Agents

- Broadspectrum sunscreens against UVA/UVB/visible light, with minimum SPF 30 (sun protection factor) should be given. It not only protects from tanning but also promotes safe sun behavior in patients. Sunscreens containing in addition, physical blockers like zinc oxide or titanium dioxide are effective. In patients with sensitive skin, the physical sunscreens are safer than chemical sunscreens.
- Tretinoin is the most useful agent for priming as it well known to accelerate healing and assist in uniform penetration of the peeling agent.
- Alpha hydroxy acid (AHA) like glycolic acid and lactic acid, cause thinning of the stratum corneum and hence enhance uniform penetration of the peeling agent. They are not very useful for PIH. They should be applied for a short duration initially, as they can cause irritant reactions.
- Hypopigmenting agents are essential in darker skin patients, to prevent PIH. Hydroquinone is the most effective agent, but can cause irritant and allergic contact dermatitis. Kojic acid, arbutin, licorice are alternative agents.

Priming Regimen

Morning: Broadspectrum sunscreen.

Evening: Glycolic acid 6 to 12% alone or in combination with hydroquinone or kojic acid.

Night: Tretinoin 0.025 to 0.05% alone or triple combination with hydroquinone and topical steroid, to prevent PIH.

Skin Preparation

Preparation are the steps involved immediately before applying the peel.

- Contact lenses should be removed.
- Patient washes the face with soap and water.
- Cleansing with alcohol.
- Degreasing with acetone. The pressure and strokes applied should be uniform to ensure an even peel.
- Chlorhexidine gluconate has been utilized, but it should preferably be avoided, due to the risk of keratitis, when used on the face.

Conclusion

The foundation of an effective and risk-free peeling procedure is based on a standardized priming regimen and skin preparation prior to peeling. Sunscreens, tretinoin, glycolic acid and hypopigmenting agents like hydroquinone are cornerstones of an effective priming regimen.

Key Points

√ Priming of the skin should be started 2 to 4 weeks before the peel.
√ Priming helps to accelerate healing, assist in uniform application of the peel, enhance penetration and reduces risk of complications. It reinforces compliance of the patient in sun protection and application of topical agents to maintain results of the peel.
√ Decreasing the incidence of PIH in dark skins is the most important factor in priming.
√ A standardized priming regimen helps to maintain and compare results.

References

1. Savant SS. Superficial and medium depth chemical peeling. In: Savant SS (Ed). Textbook of Dermatosurgery and Cosmetology, 2nd edn. ASCAD; 2005.pp.177-95.
2. Brody H. General peeling concepts. Chemical peeling and resurfacing, 2nd edn. St Louis: Mosby Year Book Inc., 1997.pp.39-72.
3. Resnik BI. The role of priming the skin for peels. In: Rubin MG (Ed). Chemical Peels. Procedures in cosmetic dermatology. Elsevier Inc. 2006.pp.21-6.
4. Hevia O, Nemeth AJ, Taylor JR. Tretinoin accelerates healing after TCA chemical peels. Arch Dermatol. 1991;127:678-82.
5. Nanda S, Grover C, Reddy BSN. Efficacy of hydroquinone (2%) versus tretinoin (0.025%) as adjunct topical agents for chemical peeling in patients of melasma. Dermatol Surg. 2004;30(3):385-9.

7

Glycolic Acid Peels

Niti Khunger

- Mechanism of Action
- Choosing a Peel Formulation
- Equipment and Reagents
- Indications
- Contraindications
- Prepeel Assessment
- Priming and Prepeel Preparation
- Procedure
- Peeling Endpoint
- Postpeel Care
- Maintenance Peels
- Complications
- Bottomline

Introduction

Alpha hydroxy acids are also called as fruit acids as they occur naturally in certain fruits, e.g. glycolic acid in sugarcane, citric acid in citrus fruits, malic acid in apples, tartaric acid in grape wine. They are the most widely used peeling agents. Alpha hydroxy acid peels are popular because they are superficial peels with a quick recovery time. Hence they are also called as 'lunchtime peels'. Glycolic acid has the smallest molecular weight of the AHA and is easily able to penetrate the skin. It is also the most scientifically studied, can be used in all skin types and is considered the gold standard of peeling agents. It is a weak acid with a pKa of 3.8.

Mechanism of Action[1]

Glycolic acid has a dual mode of action. At an acidic pH, less than the pKa, it has a keratolytic action. With a higher pH it acts as a moisturizer. It has a metabolic action and interferes with the working of enzymes such as kinases, sulfotransferases and phosphotransferases that are responsible for adhesion of the corneocytes. This causes corneocyte dysadhesion, leading to exfoliation. However, in strong concentrations, with high amount of free acid, it has a destructive effect. Since it is a weak acid, it does not have a self-neutralizing action by coagulation of proteins. It has to be neutralized by water or a weak buffer like sodium bicarbonate.

Choosing a Peel Formulation[2-4]

Glycolic acid is available as synthetic crystals dissolved in a vehicle. It may be dissolved in water or a combination of water, alcohol and propylene glycol. The peel formulation should be chosen with care as the vehicle has a key role in the concentration of free acid and efficacy of the peel. It is used as a peeling agent in a concentration of 35 to 70%. Various formulations are available.

- *Free acid:* It is a non-neutralized aqueous acidic solution with greater bioavailability of free acid and increased reactivity. Though more effective, it causes greater burning and stinging and can easily lead to epidermolysis on sensitive skins, with impaired barrier function.
- *Partially neutralized:* It is a partially neutralized form with addition of a base, ammonium hydroxide. This raises the pH of the solution, and is said to be less irritant.
- *Buffered:* It is partially neutralized stable form and has no advantage over existing solutions.
- *Esterified:* It is a solution forming glycol-citrate, which is said to be less irritant.

- *Gel based:* These are formulated in a gel base, where less free acid is available and is released slowly. It is said to be less irritant, though less efficacious and more suitable for sensitive skins.

Stability: It is stable and not light sensitive. Reagents in tightly closed bottles are stable for at least two years.

Storage: It has deliquescent properties, i.e. it absorbs moisture from the atmosphere and hence must be capped tightly.

Equipment and Reagents

- Correctly labeled glycolic acid solutions, 20%, 35%, 50%, 70%.
- Alcohol to clean the skin
- Acetone to degrease the skin
- Cold water
- Syringes filled with normal saline for irrigation of the eyes, in case of accidental spillage
- Neutralizing solutions, water or 15% sodium bicarbonate
- Glass cup or beaker in which the required agent is poured
- Head band or cap for the patient
- Gloves
- Cotton-tipped applicators or swab sticks
- 2″ × 2″ cotton gauze pieces
- Fan for cooling
- Timer.

Indications[5-11]

Since it acts mainly as a superficial peel, it is used more as a freshening peel, causing light exfoliation.
- A*esthetic:*
    - Improvement of fine lines. It is not useful in treating deep wrinkles.
    - Photoaging

- Rough textured skin.
- Reducing open skin pores
- *Pigmentation:*
  - Melasma—higher concentrations of 70% done serially, two weeks apart for at least 6 to 8 sessions. Thereafter monthly maintenance peels are needed. It should be performed with great caution in darker skins due to risk of postinflammatory hyperpigmentation (PIH) and combined with hypopigmenting agents (Figures 7.1A and B).

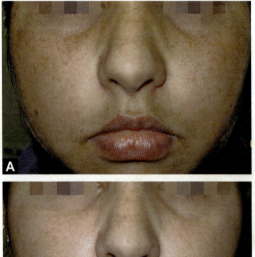

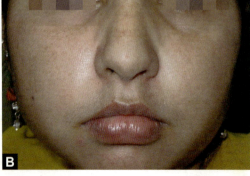

Figs 7.1A and B Melasma with lentigines treated with 2 sessions of glycolic acid 70

- – Postinflammatory hyperpigmentation (Figures 7.2A and B).
- – Freckles
- – Lentigines.
- *Acne:*
  - – Comedonal acne
  - – Pigmented acne scars
  - – Superficial depressed acne scars.
- *Keratotic lesions:*
  - – Seborrheic keratosis
  - – Dermatosis papulosa nigra
  - – *Actinic keratoses:* It may be used in combination with 5-fluorouracil. The glycolic acid facilitates penetration of 5-FU and has a synergistic effect.

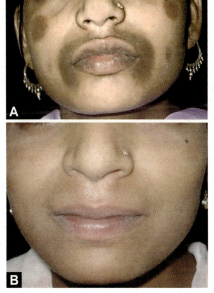

Figs 7.2A and B PIH treated with glycolic acid (GA) 6 peels every 2 weeks

-   *Keratosis pilaris:* It causes desquamation of the follicular keratotic lesion on the face, upper arms and thighs. Maintenance peels are required to prevent recurrence, which is common.
-   *Resistant warts:* It may be used for resistant warts in high concentrations, under occlusion.

The value of glycolic acid peels, even in darker skins for the treatment of melasma, PIH and acne has been well established. Grover et al.[5] used lower concentrations of glycolic acid beginning at 10% and increasing to 30% in their series of 41 patients, skin type III–V, of melasma, PIH, superficial scarring and acne. Majority of the patients had good results, and also showed improvement in texture and skin rejuvenation. There was a poor response in dermal melasma. Side effects were minimal. Burns et al.[11] also reported improvement in their dark skin patients with PIH, with minimal side effects.

A study of chemical peeling with 30% glycolic acid in a gel form was done for the treatment of open pores.[7] Peels were performed at 2 weekly intervals for two weeks. Evaluation was done using dermatoscopic analysis and an objective computerized software. Significant improvement in open pores was seen in 86% of patients with a mean improvement of 34.6% and darker pores improved in 81% of patients with a mean improvement of 34.1%. Better improvement was seen in older patients in their 40 to 60s as compared to younger patients.

Contraindications

-   Active viral, bacterial or fungal infection
-   Inflammatory dermatoses on the face
-   Patient with unrealistic expectations
-   Patients on photosensitizing drugs

- Patients who have undergone a resurfacing procedure such as dermabrasion, laser resurfacing, deep peels or any surgeries in the last 6 to 12 months.

Prepeel Assessment

A detailed history and examination is important, before peeling. Relevant history should include keloidal tendency, tendency for postinflammatory hyperpigmentation and general medical history and occupation, to judge level of sun exposure. Patients with history of herpes simplex should be put on prophylactic acyclovir 200 mg 5 times a day or famciclovir 250 mg 3 times a day, beginning two days before the peel and continued for 7 to 10 days after the peel, till complete re-epithelialization. However, prophylactic antiviral therapy is not mandatory in patients undergoing very superficial peels up to stratum corneum only, whereas it is mandatory in all patients undergoing medium and deep peels. Medications that may cause photosensitivity should ideally be stopped and alternatives given. In medium and deep peels, history of recent isotretinoin treatment in the last six months, any previous facial surgical treatment, immunocompromising conditions and smoking that may delay healing is important. This is not relevant for superficial peels. Medical examination should include general physical examination and detailed cutaneous examination. The skin type, degree of photoaging, sebaceous activity (oily or dry skin), presence of postinflammatory hyperpigmentation, presence of keloid or hypertrophic scar, presence of infection and pre-existing inflammation are important. A psychological evaluation of the patient, expected results and adequate counseling are essential to achieve a satisfactory outcome.

Priming and Prepeel Preparation

Priming at least two weeks prior to the peeling procedure is important. Dark skin patients should use a sunscreen and hypopigmenting agents, like hydroquinone or kojic acid and topical retinoid. Low concentrations of glycolic acid 6 to 12% are useful in the prepeel period and may be useful as an early indicator of patients likely to develop unusual sensitivity to glycolic acid. Some recommend a test peel in the temple or postauricular area, before peeling the full face. Cream formulations should be used for dry skins, gels for oily skins and lotions for normal skins.

All other treatments such as scrubs, microdermabrasion, depilatories, waxing, bleaching and hair removal lasers should be avoided 1 week prior to peeling. Topical retinoids should be stopped 5 to 7 days before the peel to avoid uneven peeling.

Informed consent and photographic documentation are important prerequisites. Contact lenses should be removed before the peel.

Procedure

- The patient is asked to wash the face with soap and water, to remove dirt and grime.
- The hair is pulled back with a hairband or cap.
- The patient lies down with head elevated to 45° with eyes closed.
- Inspect the skin to see that there are no abrasions or inflammation.
- Using 2″ × 2″ gauze pieces, the skin is cleaned with alcohol and then degreased with acetone.
- The peeling agent of required strength is poured in a glass beaker and neutralizing agent is also kept ready. Check the label carefully.
- It is best to start with 20 to 35% concentration in patients with thin, dry, sensitive skin and 50% in patients with normal skin. Keep a time of 3 minutes.
- Sensitive areas like the inner canthus of the eye and nasolabial folds are protected with petrolatum or vaseline.

- The timer is started and the peeling agent is then applied either with a brush or cotton tipped applicator or gauze piece. There should be no dripping of the agent.
- The chemical is applied quickly on the entire face as cosmetic units. Begin from the forehead in an upward direction, then the right cheek, nose, left cheek and chin in that order. The perioral, upper and lower eyelids, if required, are treated last. Feathering strokes are applied at the edges, to blend with surrounding skin and prevent demarcation lines.
- A cooling fan helps to reduce burning of the skin.
- Do not pass the open bottle or the soaked applicator over the eyes to avoid accidental spillage.
- Do not leave the room and watch out for redness, hot spots and epidermolysis. If this occurs, the peel should be neutralized immediately, irrespective of the time. Epidermolysis is seen as a grayish area developing, followed by blister formation. It is more common over thin skin of the eyelids.
- The peel is neutralized after set duration of time (usually 3–5 minutes). Neutralization is done with 10 to 15% sodium bicarbonate solution or neutralizing lotion or water. The advantage of sodium bicarbonate is that it is a good indicator of complete neutralization, when the fizzing stops. The disadvantage is that heat is produced due to acid-base reaction, which can be uncomfortable.
- In case of accidental spillage in the eye, it is irrigated with copius amounts of saline.
- The skin is gently dried with gauze and the patient is asked to wash with cold water till the burning subsides. The face is patted dry, but rubbing should be avoided.
- The patient then applies a sunscreen, before leaving the clinic.
- Dermatosis papulosa nigra and seborrheic keratoses can be treated with radiofrequency ablation, CO_2 laser or TCA.

However 70% glycolic acid can also be used. Here the endpoint is epidermolysis. Seventy percent GA is applied till epidermolysis occurs. It is then neutralized with saline. The surrounding normal skin must be protected with petrolatum. The patient should be warned that a scab will form which will fall off after 5 to 10 days. In dark skin patients, adequate priming is essential in these patients to prevent PIH.

- For keratosis pilaris, a sequential peel is more useful. At first, 20% salicylic acid is applied to the affected area and washed off after pseudofrosting is complete and uniform. This is then followed with glycolic acid peels 50 to 70%. The salicylic acid takes care of the inflammatory component and the glycolic acid the keratolytic component. However, maintenance peels are required as they cannot be permanently treated.

- For multiple facial planar warts 50% glycolic acid is applied and taped for 1 hour, while protecting the surrounding normal skin.[2] It is then neutralized, sunscreen is applied and the patient leaves the clinic.

Peeling Endpoint

- *Mild erythema (Pink) level 1:* Very superficial (stratum corneum)—smoothens the skin (Figure 7.3).
- *Moderate erythema (Red) level 2:* Superficial epidermal—pigmentation, removal of epidermal lesions (Figure 7.4).
- *Epidermolysis (Grayish-white) level 3:* Upper dermis—wrinkling, superficial scars, deeper peel, with increased risk of complications (Figure 7.5).
- *Blistering (vesicles) level 4:* Upper dermis—can lead to textural changes, superficial scars, pigmentary changes (Figure 7.6). It is more common in the thinner lax skin of eyelids. Hence, this thinner skin areas should be neutralized early.

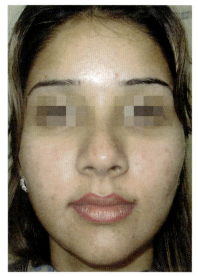

Fig. 7.3 Peeling endpoint is mild erythema

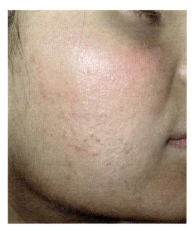

Fig. 7.4 Peeling endpoint, level 2—moderate erythema

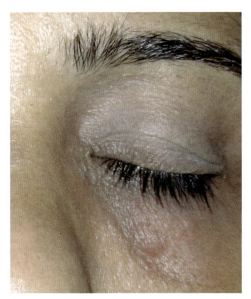

Fig. 7.5 Peeling endpoint, level 3—grayish-white appearance

However, erythema may be difficult to appreciate in dark skins, hence timing of the peel is more important.

TIMING WITH GLYCOLIC ACID PEELING (TABLE 7.1)

Sometimes erythema may be difficult to appreciate in very dark skins. Then the endpoint is judged by timing the peel.

Postpeel Care

The aim of good postoperative care is prevention, early detection and minimizing potential complications and hence ensuring early recovery of normal skin. In the postpeel period, edema, erythema and desquamation occur. In superficial peels

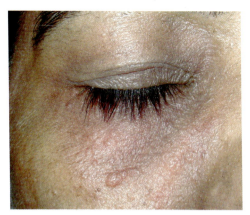

Fig. 7.6 Peeling endpoint, level 4—epidermolysis with blister formation

Table 7.1: Suggested initial timing of glycolic acid peel		
Indication	Glycolic acid %	Duration (minutes)
Acne	35–50%	1–3
Melasma	35–50%	1–3
Fine wrinkles	35–70%*	2–4
Freckles and lentigines	50–70%	3–5
Actinic/seborrheic keratoses	70%	5–7
Nonfacial	70%	5–10

Depending on skin type: 35% for thin dry skin, 70% for thick oily skin

this lasts for 1 to 3 days, whereas in deeper peels it lasts for 5 to 10 days. Mild soap or non-soap cleanser may be used. If there is crusting, topical antibacterial ointment should be used to prevent bacterial infection. Ice cold compresses or calamine lotion may be used to soothe the skin. Patients should be told to use broad-spectrum sunscreens and bland moisturizers only, till peeling is complete. Peeling or scratching the skin should be strictly avoided. Once the skin has re-epithelialized, the agents used for priming are restarted. Hypopigmenting agents are very important as PIH is very common in dark skin patients.

Maintenance Peels

Subsequently, depending on patient response, the duration of peel is increased to 5 minutes. When patient is able to tolerate, the concentration is increased to 70% for 1 to 3 minutes. Peels are repeated every 2 weeks for 12 to 16 weeks, till response. Once satisfactory response is seen, maintenance peels are done monthly for 6 months.

Complications

The best way to avoid complications is to identify patients at risk and use lighter peels. The deeper the peel, the greater is the risk of complications. Patients at risk are those with a history of postinflammatory hyperpigmentation, keloid formation, heavy occupational exposure to sun such as field workers, un-cooperative patients and patients with a history of sensitive skin unable to tolerate sunscreens, hydroquinone, etc. Such patients should be closely followed up and if complications develop, they should be treated promptly and further peels should be stopped or postponed.

- *Epidermolysis:* If it has occurred during the peel, scab formation can take place and healing is delayed. Topical moisturizer and 1% hydrocortisone is used. If severe edema occurs a short course of systemic corticosteroids, prednisolone 30 to 40 mg as a single morning dose can be given for 3 to 5 days.
- *Pigmentary changes:* Postinflammatory hyperpigmen-tation (very common) (Figure 7.7) and hypo-pigmentation

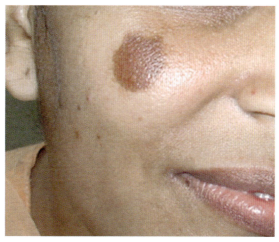

Fig. 7.7 Postinflammatory hyperpigmentation as a complication,
developing after 2 peels, with glycolic acid 70%

(rare). These can be very persistent and often difficult to
treat. They may be treated with broad spectrum sunscreens,
topical corticosteroids, tretinoin, hydroquinone or alpha-
hydroxy acids as appropriate.

- *Persistent erythema:* Erythema persisting for more than
  3 weeks after a peel is indicative of early scarring and should
  be treated with potent topical corticosteroids (Figure 7.8).
  However they should not be used for more than 2 weeks.
- *Infections:* Infections are rare with superficial peels.
  Bacterial infections can be caused *by Staphylococcus,
  Streptococcus* and *Pseudomonas.* Viral (Herpes simplex)
  and fungal (*Candida*) infections can also occur. They
  should be treated aggressively and appropriately.
- Scarring is rare in superficial peels. Proper choice of peeling
  agent, concentration and good postoperative care can help
  in prevention.
- Allergic reactions, contact urticaria.

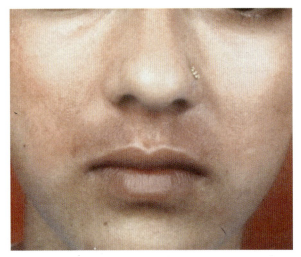

Fig. 7.8 Persistent erythema after 2 peels

- Milia
- Acneiform eruptions, particularly in the perioral area and chin.
- Lines of demarcation
- Textural changes.

Bottomline

ADVANTAGES

- Glycolic acid has a long shelf life.
- It is well tolerated.
- Does not produce systemic toxicity.
- It is an effective peeling agent even in lower concentrations.

DISADVANTAGES

- There is a great variability in reactivity and efficacy.
- It is difficult to obtain a standardized solution.
- It is sometimes difficult to judge the endpoint as there is no frosting while erythema can be hard to appreciate in dark-skinned patients.
- It has to be neutralized.
- Dermal wounds and scarring can occur in higher concentrations.
- It is expensive as compared to other peeling agents.

Conclusion

Glycolic acid peels are excellent tools for superficial chemical peeling. They are safe, with virtually no significant downtime and fit well into today's lifestyles.

Key Points

√ The efficacy of glycolic acid peels is highly dependent on the peel formulation.
√ Glycolic acid can create dermal wounds.
√ Need to be repeated for best effect.
√ Some patients improve significantly and some do not.
√ Since results are variable, do not promise a lot in the first 2 to 3 peels.

References

1. Dewandre L. The chemistry of peels and a hypothesis of action mechanisms. In: Rubin MG (Ed). Chemical peels—procedures in cosmetic dermatology. Elsevier Inc; 2006.pp.1-12.
2. Ditre CM. Alpha-hydroxy acid peels. In: Rubin MG (Ed). Chemical peels. Procedures in cosmetic dermatology. Elsevier Inc; 2011. pp.27-40.

3. Brody H. Superficial peeling. Chemical peeling and resurfacing (2nd edn). St Louis: Mosby Year Book Inc; 1997.pp.73-108.

4. Gupta RR, Mahajan BB, Garg G. Chemical peeling—evaluation of glycolic acid in varying concentrations and time intervals. Indian J Dermatol Venereol Leprol. 2001;67:28-9.

5. Grover C, Reddu BS. The therapeutic value of glycolic acid peels in dermatology. Indian J Dermatol Venereol Leprol. 2003;69(2):148-50.

6. Sarkar R, Kaur C, Bhalla M, et al. The combination of glycolic acid peels with a topical regimen in the treatment of melasma in dark-skinned patients: A comparative study. Dermatol Surg 2002;28(9):828-32;discussion 832.

7. Kakudo N, Kushida S, Tanaka N, Minakata T, Suzuki K, Kusumoto K. A novel method to measure conspicuous facial pores using computer analysis of digital-camera-captured images: the effect of glycolic acid chemical peeling. Skin Res Technol. 2011;17:427-33.

8. Atzori L, Brundu MA, Orru A, et al. Glycolic acid peeling in the treatment of acne. J Eur Acad Dermatol Venereol. 1999;12(2):119-22.

9. Javaheri SM, Handa S, Kaur I, et al. Safety and efficacy of glycolic acid facial peel in Indian women with melasma. Int J Dermatol 2001;40(5):354-7.

10. Erbil H, Sezer E, Taştan B, et al. Efficacy and safety of serial glycolic acid peels and a topical regimen in the treatment of recalcitrant melasma. J Dermatol. 2007;34(1):25-30.

11. Burns RL, Prevost-Blank PL, Lawry MA, et al. Glycolic acid peels for postinflammatory hyperpigmentation in black patients. A comparative study. Dermatol Surg. 1997;23(3):171-4; discussion 175.

8

Trichloroacetic Acid Peels

Niti Khunger

- Mechanism of Action
- Peel Formulation
- Equipment and Reagents
- Superficial Peels
- Priming and Prepeel Preparation
- Procedure for Superficial Peels
- Procedure for Medium Depth Peels
- Postpeel Care
- Complications
- TCA CROSS (Chemical Reconstruction of Skin Scars) Technique for Icepick Scars
- Bottomline
- TCA with Sand Abrasion for Acne Scars

Introduction

Trichloroacetic acid (TCA) is a common peeling agent used for superficial as well as medium depth peels. It is a versatile peeling agent, since the peel depth can be varied according to the concentration of the solution (Table 8.1). TCA was first employed as a peeling agent by Unna, a German dermatologist in 1882. Since then there have been numerous reports on the use of TCA for superficial as well as medium depth peels.[1]

Table 8.1: Depth of trichloroacetic acid (TCA) peel according to concentration	
Concentration of TCA	Peel depth
10–15%	Very superficial
15–25%	Superficial
35–50%	Medium depth

Mechanism of Action[2]

It is caustic and causes coagulation of skin proteins leading to frosting. Precipitation of proteins leads to necrosis and destruction of the epidermis. The depth of destruction depends on the concentration of TCA. The higher the concentration, the deeper is the penetration; hence it has a predictable effect. Coagulation is followed by inflammation and activation of mechanisms of wound repair. This leads to re-epithelialization, with replacement of smoother skin, with an even skin tone. In addition, in medium depth peels there is collagen remodeling, with production of new collagen in the dermis. It is self-neutralizing and hence not absorbed in the systemic circulation.

Peel Formulation

Trichloroacetic acid (TCA) is available as anhydrous, hygroscopic white crystals, which are dissolved in distilled water to make a solution. Its molecular structure is close to glycolic acid. It is a stronger acid with pKa value of 0.26. Various strengths can be prepared and stored in glass bottles. It has deliquescent properties and hence old crystals that are exposed to air should not be used. The safe peeling concentration begins with 10%, which may go up to 25%. Higher concentrations of 35% create deeper peels and should be avoided in dark skins. Concentrations above 35% have a high risk of causing textural changes and scarring and should be avoided in all skin types. If deeper penetration is required, lower concentrations, 15 to 25% can be combined with other peeling agents or other modalities.

Fresh solutions should be prepared every 6 months.

- Trichloroacetic acid (TCA) solution 15% W/V. TCA USP crystals 15 gm, distilled water add to make 100 mL. Some add 10 mL glycerine with distilled water to make 100 mL.
- Easy TCA® (Skintech), Obagi blue peel® (TCA is the active ingredient mixed with the patented Blue Base, for easy visualization), Accupeel® (TCA Mask, 11% or 16% in a cream formulation) are some patented formulations available.

Storage: Store in glass bottles. Not light sensitive. Refrigeration is not needed.

Stability: Stable for at least 6 months. Solution should be clear, colorless and free of any particles.

Equipment and Reagents

- TCA solutions 10%, 15%, 25%, for superficial peels. TCA 35% for medium peels, but use with caution in skin types IV to VI. It is better to combine two peeling agents in lower concentrations, to increase depth of the peel. In darker skins, it is advisable not to exceed a concentration of 25% TCA.
- Alcohol to clean the skin.
- Acetone to degrease the skin.
- Spray of cold water.
- Petrolatum or vaseline® to protect sensitive areas.
- Syringes filled with normal saline for irrigation of eyes, in case of accidental spillage.
- Glass cup or beaker in which the peeling agent is poured.
- Cotton tipped applicators or swab sticks.
- 2″ × 2″ cotton gauze pieces.
- Gloves.
- Head band or cap for the patient.
- Fan for cooling.

Superficial Peels

INDICATIONS[3-6]

Photoaging

- Fine few wrinkles
- Dyschromias.

Textural Changes

- Oily skin
- Rough uneven skin
- Dilated pores.

Hyperpigmentation

- Epidermal melasma (Figure 8.1)
- Postinflammatory hyperpigmentation
- Freckles
- Lentigines.

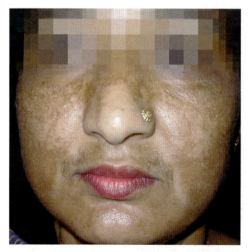

Fig. 8.1 Epidermal melasma

Acne

- Pigmented acne scars
- Superficial mild acne scars.

CONTRAINDICATIONS

- Active bacterial infection in the area to be peeled.
- Active herpes simplex.
- Viral warts or molluscum contagiosum on the area to be peeled.
- Open wounds, inflammation or irritation.
- History of taking photosensitive drugs.
- Uncooperative patient, e.g. patient is careless about sun exposure or application of medicine as directed.
- Patient with unrealistic expectations.

Priming and Prepeel Preparation

For superficial peels, priming at least 2 weeks and preferably 4 weeks in darker skins, prior to the peeling procedure is important. Dark skin patients should use a broad-spectrum sunscreen protecting against ultraviolet A (UVA) and ultraviolet B (UVB) and in addition minimize sun exposure by physical methods such as umbrellas or hats. Hypopigmenting agents, like hydroquinone 2 to 5%, kojic acid 1 to 2% and topical retinoids are essential as postinflammatory hyperpigmentation (PIH) is very common with TCA peels. Low concentrations of glycolic acid 6 to 12% are useful in the prepeel period, particularly in patients with thick, oily skins. Priming gives an early indication of patients likely to develop unusual sensitivity to the sunscreen, hydroquinone or glycolic acid. Some recommend a test peel in the temple or postauricular area, 2 weeks before peeling the full face. This is important in patients with sensitive skins. Cream formulations should be used for dry skins, gels for oily skins and lotions for normal skins.

All other treatments such as scrubs, microdermabrasion, depilatories, waxing, bleaching and hair removal lasers should be avoided 1 week prior to peeling. Topical retinoids should be stopped 5 to 7 days before the peel to avoid uneven peeling.

Informed consent and photographic documentation are important prerequisites. Contact lenses should be removed before the peel.

Procedure for Superficial Peels

- The patient is asked to wash the face with soap and water to remove dust and grime.
- The hair is pulled back with a hairband or cap.
- The patient lies down with head elevated to 450 with eyes closed.
- Using 2″ × 2″ gauze pieces, the skin is cleaned with alcohol and then degreased with acetone or a prepeel cleanser which accompanies the kit. Cleaning should not be vigorous, particularly in patients with thin dry skin as it can increase the depth of the peel.
- Sensitive areas of the face such as the lips, inner canthus of the eye and the nasolabial folds are protected with a thin layer of petrolatum.
- TCA 10 to 15% is used for very superficial peels (up to stratum corneum). TCA 25% is used for superficial peels (up to basal layer of epidermis). Dark skin patients often react unpredictably to TCA peels; hence it is advised to use a lower concentration of 10% if the skin is thin and dry and 15% for normal skin, when peeling the patient for the first time.
- The peeling agent of the desired concentration is then applied either with a brush or cotton tipped applicator or gauze piece. There should be no dripping of the agent and the applicator should not pass across the eyes.
- The chemical is applied quickly on the entire face as separate cosmetic units. Begin from the forehead in an upward direction, then the nose and pause to observe the nature of frost developing. Then apply on the right cheek,

left cheek and chin in that order. The perioral, upper and lower eyelids, if required, are treated last. The skin should be stretched when applying in areas of wrinkling so that the acid reaches the bottom of the wrinkle or line. Care should be taken that the acid does not reach the eye and the skin should be held taught till the acid dries and frosting is complete. Feathering strokes are applied at the edges, to blend with the hairline and surrounding skin to prevent demarcation lines.

- A cooling fan helps to reduce burning of the skin.

PEELING END POINT

- In a very superficial peel, no frosting or very minute speckles of frost may be seen. The skin looks shiny, with minimal or no erythema (Level 0).
- In a superficial peel, involving the epidermis partially, frosting is scattered, light white with mild erythema. This peel will flake lightly and heal in 2 to 4 days (Level 1) (Figure 8.2).

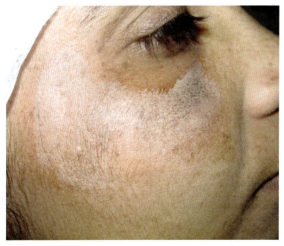

Fig. 8.2 Frosting level 1 scattered light white frost, 15% TCA

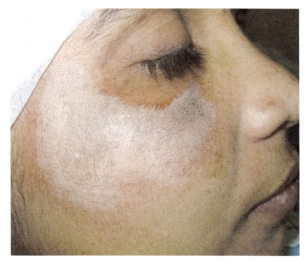

Fig. 8.3 Frosting level 2, speckled white frost, 25% TCA

- Where a little deeper peeling is required, a second coat is applied a little vigorously to get a speckled whiter frost with erythema showing through (Level 2) (Figure 8.3). This implies a superficial full thickness epidermal peel that may take 5 to 7 days to heal. A solid white frost indicates a deeper medium depth peel up to papillary dermis and should be avoided (Level 3) (Figure 8.4).
- Once the appropriate level of frosting has occurred it is gently wiped with saline gauze to remove excess acid.
- In case of accidental spillage in the eye, it is irrigated with copious amounts of saline.
- The skin is gently dried with gauze and the patient is asked to wash with cold water till the burning subsides. The face is patted dry, but rubbing should be avoided.
- The patient then applies a sunscreen, before leaving the clinic.

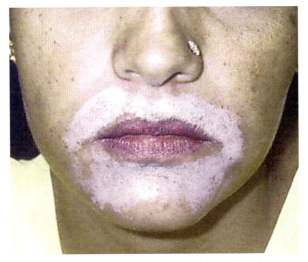

Fig. 8.4 Frosting level 3, solid white frost, 35% TCA

POSTPEEL CARE

Patients feel tightness of the skin after a peel. Sunscreens and moisturizers are used postpeel till desquamation subsides. In a very superficial peel little or no peeling may occur and skin quickly returns to normal, looking little fresh and smooth. In a superficial peel flaking occurs and scaling at few places. The skin may darken at places in darker skins, alarming the patient. However, it usually returns to normal in 2 to 7 days. Mild soap or nonsoap cleanser may be used. If there is crusting, topical antibacterial ointment should be used to prevent bacterial infection. Patients should avoid peeling or scratching the skin.

The topical skin regimen of hypopigmenting agents, acne medications, glycolic acid and retinoids is then resumed as appropriate after peeling subsides, till the next peel. Peels can be repeated every 2 weeks, till satisfactory improvement. This usually occurs after 4 to 6 peels. Maintenance peels once a month or as and when required can be done thereafter.

The TCA 3.75% and lactic acid 15% were used as a combination peel for periorbital dark circles, weekly for 4 weeks. A significant esthetic response was seen in 93.3% of the patients as assessed by a physician, whereas patient's global assessment rated as fair, good, or excellent response in 96.7% of the patients. Mild and temporary adverse effects, such as erythema, edema, frosting, dryness, and telangiectasias occured. The effects of treatment remained for at least 4 to 6 months in the majority of patients with appropriate sun protection.

MEDIUM DEPTH PEELS[7–9]

Indications

Photoaging
- Fine wrinkling, present at rest
- Seborrheic keratosis
- Dermatoses papulosa nigra.

Textural changes
- Rough uneven skin
- Dilated pores.

Hyperpigmentation
- Dermal melasma (With extreme precautions)
- Postinflammatory hyperpigmentation
- Lentigines.

Acne
- Pigmented acne scars
- Superficial acne scars.

Keratotic lesions
- Keratosis pilaris
- Warts (Figures 8.5A and B)
- Xanthelasma palpebrarum.

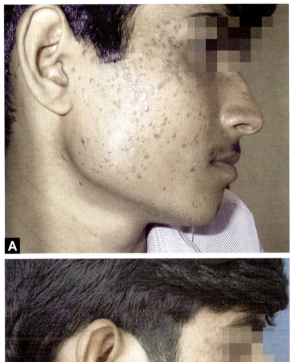

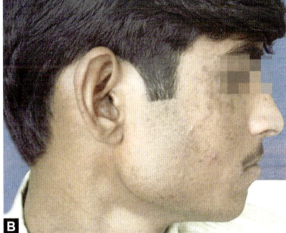

Figs 8.5A and B Warts treated with 25% TCA,
2 sittings at weekly intervals

CONTRAINDICATIONS

Medium peels should be done cautiously in dark skin patients, due to the risk of pigmentary changes.

- Active bacterial, viral infection in the area to be peeled.
- Active herpes simplex.
- Open wounds, inflammation or irritation.
- History of taking photosensitive drugs.
- Uncooperative patient, e.g. patient is careless about sun exposure or application of medicine as directed.
- Patient with unrealistic expectations.
- History of abnormal scarring such as hypertrophic scars and keloids. Examine old scars and be cautious in patients with family history of keloids.
- Atrophic skin or recent facial surgical procedures, within the last 6 months such as resurfacing, grafts, flaps, etc. which may have compromised circulation and delayed healing.
- Immunocompromised patients with delayed healing
- Isotretinoin use in the last six months.[10]

PRIMING AND PREPEEL PREPARATION

For medium depth peels, priming should be started at least 6 weeks before the procedure in skin of color. Dark skin patients should use a broad-spectrum sunscreen protecting against UVA and UVB or preferably a sunblock contain zinc oxide or titanium dioxide, and in addition minimize sun exposure by physical methods such as umbrellas. Hypopigmenting agents, like hydroquinone 2 to 5%, kojic acid 1 to 2% and topical retinoids are essential as PIH is very common with TCA peels. Low concentrations of glycolic acid 6 to 12% are useful in the prepeel period, particularly in patients with thick, oily skins. A test peel in the temple or postauricular area should be done, 2 weeks before peeling the full face. This is important in patients with sensitive skins. Cream formulations should be used for dry skins, gels for oily skins and lotions for normal skins.

Antivirals, valacyclovir 500 to 1000 mg three times a day or famciclovir 250 to 500 mg twice a day is started on the day of the procedure and continued for 5 to 7 days till healing is complete. Prednisolone 30 mg is also started on the day of the procedure and continued for 5 days, to reduce postpeel edema and inflammation.

A mild sedative like diazepam 5 mg or lorazepam 1 to 2 mg may be given in anxious patients, the night before and on the day of the peel.

All other treatments such as scrubs, microdermabrasion, depilatories, waxing, bleaching and hair removal lasers should be avoided 1 week prior to peeling. Topical retinoids should be stopped 5 to 7 days before the peel to avoid uneven peeling.

Informed consent and photographic documentation are important prerequisites. Contact lenses should be removed before the peel.

Procedure for Medium Depth Peels

- As for superficial peels, the patient is asked to wash the face with soap and water to remove dust and grime.
- The hair is pulled back with a hairband or cap.
- The patient lies down with head elevated to 45° with eyes closed.
- Using 2″ × 2″ gauze pieces, the skin is cleaned with alcohol and then degreased with acetone or a prepeel cleanser which accompanies the kit. The cleaning is done a little more vigorously, especially in thick oily skins and areas of uneven thicker texture.
- TCA 35% is applied quickly using a cotton tipped applicator on the entire face as separate cosmetic units, similar to the procedure for superficial peels.
- Frosting should be white and even, with background erythema (Level 3).
- Delicate areas such as eyelids, mandibular areas and chin should be treated cautiously as they are prone to scarring and preferably peeled with a lower concentration.

- The skin should be stretched when applying in areas of wrinkling so that the acid reaches the bottom of the wrinkle or line. Precautions should be taken so that the acid does not reach the eye and the skin should be held taut till the acid dries and frosting is complete. Dry cotton tip applicators should be held at the inner and outer canthi of the eyes to absorb tears. Feathering strokes are applied at the edges, to blend with the hairline and surrounding skin to prevent demarcation lines.
- A cooling fan helps to reduce burning of the skin. As soon as frosting is complete, cold compresses should be applied to reduce discomfort.
- The patient is then asked to wash the face repeatedly with water till the burning subsides. This also helps in reducing the frost so that patient can leave the clinic early.
- A sunscreen is applied before leaving the clinic.

Postpeel Care

The patient should be adequately informed about the sequence of events after a medium peel and how to take good care so as to reduce the chances of complications. Initially, the skin will look and feel tight. Swelling around the eyes is common, that peaks in 2 to 3 days and subsides in 4 to 5 days. Oral prednisolone 30 mg given for 5 days greatly helps in reducing edema. Any area of hyperpigmentation and scaling will show increased pigmentation that can alarm the patient. This is more conspicuous in darker skins and is part of normal peeling reaction. Bland moisturizers are liberally applied to reduce discomfort and cracking. Mild soap or non-soap cleanser may be used. They should be gently applied, washed off and the face patted gently.

The skin then begins to crack and peel, initially at sites of muscle movement such as the perioral areas and cheeks. The forehead and hairline and sides of the face are the last to peel. If there is crusting, topical antibacterial ointment like mupirocin 2% ointment should be used to prevent bacterial infection. Patients should avoid peeling or scratching or rubbing the skin. Premature peeling and picking the skin, exposes the underlying new skin and increases risk of infection, persistent erythema, hyperpigmentation and scarring. Itching is common as the skin heals and topical 1% hydrocortisone is useful if it is severe.

The skin gradually peels off and re-epithelialization is complete in 7 to 10 days. Light make up can now be applied to cover erythema and patient can join work, taking strict precautions with sun exposure. Sunscreens should be repeatedly and generously applied every 2 to 3 hours as this is the time when postinflammatory hyperpigmentation can set in, particulary in darker skin types. Antivirals can be stopped. Erythema gradually fades in 2 to 3 weeks. Rarely, it may be persistent beyond 4 weeks. Topical hydrocortisone 1% is used, if this occurs.

If healing is delayed beyond 10 days, it is a sign of infection, bacterial, viral or fungal or irritant contact reaction and should be treated appropriately.

Pretreatment priming agents are then restarted, particularly the hypopigmenting agents, to prevent PIH. The skin may feel sensitive postpeel and lower strengths of retinoids or glycolic acid should be used.

Medium peels should not be repeated before 6 months, if required, preferably after 1 year.

NONFACIAL TRICHLOROACETIC ACID PEELS[11]

Medium peels should preferably be avoided with TCA in nonfacial areas due to risk of delayed healing and increased complications. Repeated superficial peels are efficacious in removing pigmentary changes and mild wrinkling.

COMBINATION PEELS AND PROCEDURES

TCA beyond 35% greatly increases the risk of scarring. In order to increase the depth of the peel, without increasing concentration of TCA beyond 35%, combination peels were introduced (For details see Chapter 15)

- Solid CO_2 and TCA 35% (Brody's peel)[12]
- Glycolic acid 70% and TCA 35% (Coleman's peel)[13]
- Jessner's solution and TCA 35% (Monheit's peel)[14]
- Sand abrasion and TCA 15 to 25%. This is useful for darker and sensitive skins.[15–17] (Figures 8.6 and 8.7).
- CO_2 laser and TCA 35%[18]

All combinations therapies utilizing concentration of TCA beyond 25% should be avoided in darker skin types.

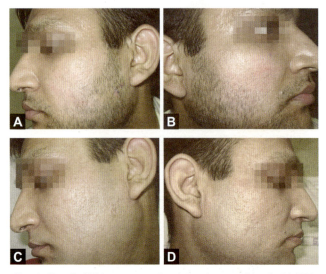

Figs 8.6A to D Mild acne scars, Sand abrasion, combined with TCA 15%. (A and B) Before treatment; (C and D) After treatment

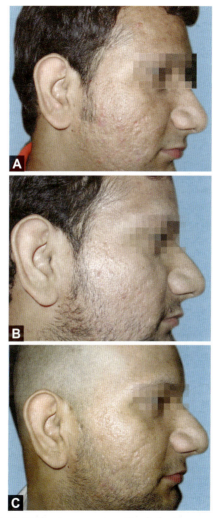

Figs 8.7A to C Moderate acne scars, Sand abrasion, combined with TCA 15%. (A) Before treatment; (B) 2 months after 1 session; (C) After 6 months

Complications[19,20]

The best way to avoid complications is to identify patients at risk and use lighter peels. The deeper the peel, the greater is the risk of complications. Medium peels should be avoided or done with great precaution in type IV to VI skins. Patients at risk are those with a history of postinflammatory hyperpigmentation, keloid formation, heavy occupational exposure to sun such as field workers, uncooperative patients and patients with a history of sensitive skin unable to tolerate sunscreens, hydroquinone, etc. Such patients should be closely followed up and if complications develop, they should be treated promptly and further peels should be stopped or postponed.

COMPLICATIONS OF SUPERFICIAL PEELS

- Edema
- Severe pain and burning
- Persistent erythema
- Pruritus
- Bacterial infection
- Herpetic infection
- Candidal infection
- Hyperpigmentation
- Hypopigmentation
- Demarcation lines
- Ocular complications
- Acneiform eruptions
- Allergic reactions
- Scarring.

COMPLICATIONS OF MEDIUM PEELS

In addition to complications of superficial peels:
- Premature peeling
- Infection

- Persistent erythema
- Hyperpigmentation
- Hypopigmentation
- Scarring
- Milia
- Delayed healing
- Textural changes.

BACTERIAL INFECTION

Infections are uncommon with superficial peels, but can occur in hot humid climates with excessive sweating. They can occur in medium peels due to delayed healing and premature peeling of the skin. Infection should be suspected when there is oozing, crusting and delayed healing. Suspected infections should be treated aggressively to prevent scarring and PIH. A Gram's stain should be done, which can detect gram-positive or gram-negative organisms or *Candida*. Swab for culture and sensitivity should be taken from a suspicious area and topical and systemic antibiotics started immediately. Impetigo and folliculitis can occur due to staphylococci and should be appropriately treated with cloxacillin or amoxycillin-clavulanic acid combination. *Streptococcus* and *Pseudomonas* infections can also occur and should be treated with appropriate antibiotics. Topical wound care is important. Wound should be cleaned 3 to 4 times a day with potassium permanganate soaks 1:10,000 (light pink color solution) or dilute acetic acid 0.25% compresses. Topical mupirocin ointment for gram-positive organisms should be used.

HERPETIC INFECTION

This can be triggered by a medium chemical peel and rarely by a superficial peel. They usually present as painful erosions around the vermilion border of the lips. In fact, it is a cardinal principle that any painful eruption should be taken as herpes and treated likewise. If patients are already on prophylactic antiviral and herpes still occurs the dosage should be doubled.

CANDIDAL INFECTION

Candidal infection presents as superficial pustules and erosions. Patients may have angular cheilitis or oral thrush. Gram's stain reveals the diagnosis. They should be treated with fluconazole 50 mg or ketoconazole 200 mg per day, along with topical clotrimazole 1% cream.

HYPERPIGMENTATION (FIGURES 8.8A AND B)

Hyperpigmentation is very common, in patients with skin types III to VI undergoing superficial or medium peels. It can occur anytime after the peel and can be persistent, if inadequately treated. Hence, it is important to educate the patient about avoiding sun exposure and use of broad-spectrum sunscreens before and indefinitely after the peels. Hyperpigmentation can also occur in patients using photosensitizing drugs such as nonsteroidal anti-inflammatory drugs (NSAIDs), oral contraceptives (OC), etc. Hyperpigmentation can also occur in type I to II skins following intense sun exposure and tanning or use of photosensitizing agents.

Priming the patient with suitable topical hypopigmenting agents such as hydroquinone, kojic acid, arbutin, etc. is an important part of the peeling regimen and should be strictly enforced in the postpeel period. When hyperpigmentation occurs, triple combinations of hydroquinone, tretinoin and steroids are useful and are restarted once re-epithelialization is complete.

HYPOPIGMENTATION (FIGURE 8.9)

A lighter and fairer complexion is normally seen after peeling and in fact may be the desired result in darker skins, who

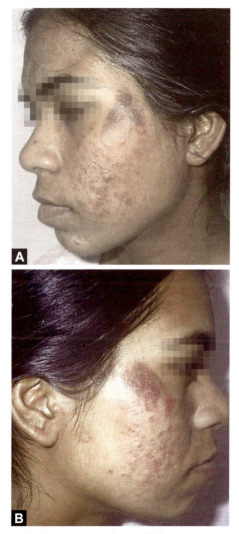

Figs 8.8A and B Complication of superficial peel hyperpigmentation

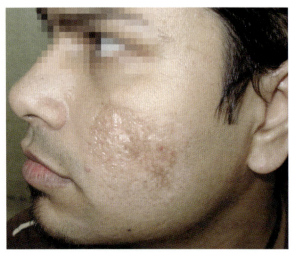

Fig. 8.9 Complication of medium depth peel, hypopigmentation and hyperpigmentation

strongly desire a fairer complexion. This effect is transient in superficial peels and occurs due to sloughing off of the epidermis and removal of excess melanin. In medium peels, with removal of the basal layer, the hypopigmentation can be more prolonged, till melanocytes migrate from the surrounding skin and adnexae. In darker skins this hypopigmentation can be followed by PIH, due to overactivity of the melanocytes, hence medium peels are done with great caution in darker individuals.

LINES OF DEMARCATION (FIGURE 8.10)

These are lines of pigmentary change at the junction of peeled and unpeeled areas. They are common in all skin types and more common in darker skins and medium and deep peels. The periocular, perioral and jaw line are common

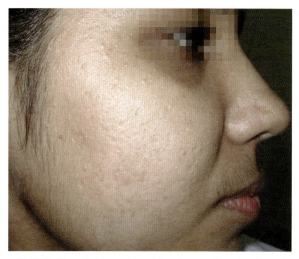

Fig. 8.10 Line of demarcation following medium depth peel

sites of predilection. To avoid this, peeling agent with a lower concentration should be feathered at the edges to merge with the surrounding normal skin.

SCARRING

Scarring is uncommon with superficial peels, but more common with medium peels and very common if TCA concentration exceeds 50%. Sites prone to scarring are the temple and mandibular area and perioral region. Patients developing reactions, infections and premature peeling are at increased risk for scarring. Scars can be flat hypopigmented and shiny with loss of texture or depressed atrophic with sharp demarcation. Thickened, hypertrophic keloidal scarring can occur in prone individuals with medium peels, especially over the jaw area. Hypertrophic scars should be treated with potent topical steroids, clobetasol proprionate for 2 weeks followed by mometasone till erythema and induration disappear. The pulsed dye laser may also be useful in treating incipient scarring and reducing erythema.

MILIA

Milia are not seen in superficial peels but can occur in medium peels, 2 to 3 weeks after peeling. They usually subside spontaneously or can be extracted with a 26 gauge needle.

DELAYED HEALING

It is more common in medium peels and in nonfacial areas, particularly in smokers, immunocompromised patients and those with previous facial surgery and radiation. Delayed healing can occur due to infection, irritation, premature peeling, in patients who have undergone previous facial surgery, radiation or in immunocompromised states. Aggressive wound care management is important to prevent infection and scarring. Topical mupirocin ointment along with systemic antibiotics with good coverage of staphylococci should be given till re-epithelialization is complete.

TEXTURAL CHANGES

Textural changes can occur due to uneven peel depth. Products that peel the skin such as tretinoin, glycolic acid and scrubs should be stopped 2 to 3 days before peeling. Degreasing the skin and application of the peel should be uniform. Textural changes may improve by repeeling after 3 months.

SPOT PEELS[21]

Spot peels are peels limited to the affected area only. They are indicated when there are few or localized lesions. Freckles, lentigines, postinflammatory hyperpigmentation, seborrheic

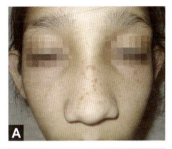
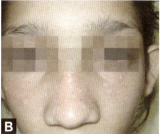
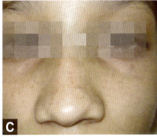

Figs 8.11A to C Spot peels, freckles, 25% TCA after 1 peel. (A) Freckles before treatment; (B) Frosting after application of 25% TCA; (C) After 1 session

and actinic keratoses, dermatosis papulosa nigra, localized superficial acne scars, fixed drug eruption, etc. can be safely treated by spot peels (Figures 8.11 and 8.12).

The concentrations that can be used safely for some common conditions are as follows:

- Freckles, lentigines, PIH, FDE—15 to 30%
- Superficial acne scars—30 to 50%
- DPN, seborrheic and actinic keratoses, skin tags—30 to 50%
- Warts Molluscum contagiosum—50 to 70%

The chemical is applied with a tooth pick or pointed swab stick on the lesion. The surrounding normal skin is protected with an occlusive ointment such as paraffin. The advantage of spot peeling is that the entire normal area is spared, hence healing is faster and the risk of complications is lower. This is particularly important in skin of color where higher concentrations can easily lead to pigmentary changes. In

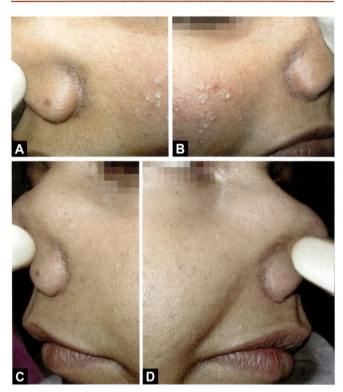

Figs 8.12A to D Spots peel, seborrheic melanosis, 50% TCA, after 1 peel

addition, since only the lesion is targeted, higher concentrations can be safely used.

TCA CROSS (Chemical Reconstruction of Skin Scars) Technique for Icepick Scars[22,23]

Trichloroacetic acid in high concentration (50%, 65%, 100%) causes full thickness skin necrosis. This is used to destroy the tract of the icepick scar. Subsequent collagen deposition fills the depressed icepick scar. No local anesthesia is required. After cleaning and degreasing the skin, the acid is carefully applied within the scar only, without spillage on the surrounding skin. It is best done using a fine pointed sterile wooden tip of a toothpick. The treated scar immediately blanches with an intense white frost, due to coagulation of epidermal and dermal proteins. An antibiotic based ointment like mupirocin is applied. Within 1 to 3 days crusts are formed, which fall off in 3 to 5 days. Collagen formation causes elevation of the scar. This may take 2 to 3 weeks and can continue up to 4 to 6 weeks. A sunscreen is applied during the day and 0.05% tretinoin and 5% hydroquinone cream is applied at night for a minimum of 4 weeks, to prevent postinflammatory hyperpigmentation. On an average about 25% improvement of scars takes place with 1 sitting. The procedure may be repeated 2 or 3 times, at intervals of 1 to 3 months for full elevation. It then can be combined with other resurfacing procedures to correct the other types of scars. The advantage of the chemical reconstruction of skin scars (CROSS) technique is that since the adjacent normal tissue and adnexal structures are spared, healing is more rapid with a lower complication rate than conventional full-face medium to deep chemical resurfacing. However, PIH is very common in patients with darker skins, which may be prolonged. Hence, the patient should be primed adequately with hypopigmenting agents prior to the procedure and these should be continued till improvement (Figures 8.13A to H).

Bottomline

ADVANTAGES OF TCA

- Stable
- No systemic toxicity
- The peel depth correlates with the intensity of the frost
- The end point is easy to judge

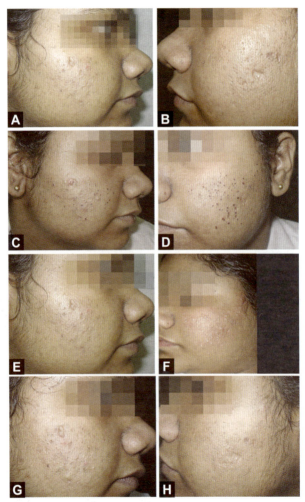

Figs 8.13A to H Icepick acne scars, CROSS technique, 50% TCA. (A and B) Before treatment; (C and D) Frosting after application of 50% TCA; (E and F) Skin necrosis at third day; (G and H) Healing after 7 days

- No need of neutralization
- TCA is easily available
- Easy to prepare
- It is inexpensive.

DISADVANTAGES OF TCA

- More prone to cause PIH in darker skins.
- Higher concentrations 35% and above can cause scarring.

TCA with Sand Abrasion for Acne Scars (see Chapter 16)

In sand abrasion, sterile sandpaper is used to abrade the skin, up to a level of the papillary dermis. This is followed by chemical peeling with 10 to 15% TCA. The advantage is that a greater depth of peeling is possible, without increasing the concentration of TCA. Secondly, sandpaper abrasion is not very uniform and hence leaves minute islands of normal skin, hence re-epithelialization is quicker, with a reduced downtime. Since lower concentrations of peeling agents are used, pigmentary changes are less common and improve faster, particularly in darker skin types.

Conclusion

TCA is a versatile peeling agent and is useful for superficial and medium peels. The results are predictable and the end point is easy to judge as the intensity of frosting correlates with peel depth. However, concentrations beyond 25% should be used cautiously in darker skins. Spot peels for localized lesions and CROSS technique for icepick scars are effective and safe for darker skins.

> **Key Points**
>
> √ Trichloroacetic acid is a versatile peeling agent and can be used for superficial as well as medium depth peels. The depth of the peel correlates with the concentration.
> √ In dark skins, 10 to 15% is a safe concentration, but concentration beyond 25% have a higher risk of pigmentary changes. It is safer to combine two peeling agents in lower concentrations sequentially rather than increase the concentration. TCA can also be combined with other techniques such as manual dermasanding.
> √ CROSS technique is useful for postacne icepick scars.

References

1. Brody H. History of Chemical peels. In: Baxter S (Ed). Chemical Peeling and Resurfacing, 2nd edn. St. Louis: Mosby Year Book Inc., 1997.pp. 1-5.
2. Dewandre L. The chemistry of peels and a hypothesis of action mechanisms. In: Rubin MG (Ed). Chemical Peels. Procedures in Cosmetic Dermatology. Elsevier Inc. 2006.pp.1-12.
3. Savant SS. Superficial and medium depth chemical peeling. In: Savant SS (Ed). Textbook of Dermatosurgery and Cosmetology, 2nd edn. ASCAD, 2005.pp.177-95.
4. Chun EY, Lee JB, Lee KH. Focal trichloroacetic acid peel method for benign pigmented lesions in dark-skinned Patients. Dermatol Surg. 2004;30:512-6.
5. Rubin MG. Trichloroacetic acid peels. In: Rubin MG (Ed). Manual of Chemical Peels-Superfical and Medium Depth, Ist edn. Philadelphia. JB Lippincot Co., 1995.pp.110-29.
6. Soliman MM, Ramadan SA, Bassiouny DA, et al. Combined trichloroacetic acid peel and topical ascorbic acid versus trichloroacetic acid peel alone in the treatment of melasma: A comparative study. J Cosmet Dermatol. 2007;6(2):89-94.
7. Vavouli C[1], Katsambas A, Gregoriou S, Teodor A, Salavastru C, Alexandru A, Kontochristopoulos G. Chemical peeling with trichloroacetic acid and lactic acid for infraorbital dark circles. J Cosmet Dermatol. 2013;12:204-9.

8. Al-Waiz MM, Al-Sharqi AI. Medium-depth chemical peels in the treatment of acne scars in dark-skinned individuals. Dermatol Surg. 2002;28(5):383-7.

9. Kadhim KA, Al-Waiz M. Treatment of periorbital wrinkles by repeated medium-depth chemical peels in dark-skinned individuals. J Cosmet Dermatol. 2005;4(1):18-22.

10. Roenigk RK. Retinoids, dermabrasion, chemical peel and keloids. In: Roenigk RK, Roenigk HH Jr (Eds). Surgical Dermatology: Advances in Current Practice. St Louis: Mosby, 1993.pp.376-83.

11. Cook KK, Cook WR Jr. Chemical peel of nonfacial skin using glycolic acid gel augmented with TCA and neutralized based on visual staging. Dermatol Surg. 2000;26(11):994-9.

12. Brody HJ, Hailey CW. Medium depth chemical peeling of the skin: A variation of superficial chemosurgery. J Derm Surg Oncol. 1986;12:1268.

13. Coleman WP III, Futrell JM. The glycolic, trichloroacetic acid peel. J Dermatol Surg Oncol. 1994;20:76-80.

14. Monheit GD. The Jessner's + TCA peel: A medium-depth chemical peel. J Dermatol Surg Oncol. 1989;15:953-63.

15. Monheit GD. Combinations of therapy. Chemical peels. In: Rubin MG (Ed). Chemical Peels. Procedures in Cosmetic Dermatology. Elsevier Inc., 2006.pp.115-36.

16. Harris DR, Noodleman FR. Combining manual dermasanding with low strength trichloroacetic acid to improve actinically injured skin. J Dermatol Surg Oncol. 1994;20:436-42.

17. Cooley JE, Casey DL, Kauffman CL. Manual resurfacing and trichloroacetic acid for the treatment of patients with widespread actinic damage. Clinical and histologic observations. Dermatol Surg. 1997;23(5):373.

18. Fulton JE, Rahimi D, Helton P, Dahlberg K. Neck rejuvenation by combining Jessner/TCA peel, dermasanding, and CO_2 laser resurfacing. Dermatol Surg. 1999;25:745-50.

19. Duffy DM. Avoiding complications with chemical peels. In: Rubin MG (Ed). Chemical Peels. Procedures in Cosmetic Dermatology. Elsevier Inc. 2006.pp.137-70.

20. Brody HJ. Complications of chemical peels. Chemical Peeling and Resurfacing, 2nd edn. Mosby Year Book Inc., 1997.pp.162-94.

21. Fung JF, Sengelmann RD, Kenneally CZ. Chemical injury to the eye from trichloroacetic acid. Dermatol Surg. 2002;28(7):609-10; discussion 610.

22. Lee JB, Chung WG, Kwahck H, Lee KH. Focal treatment of acne scars with trichloroacetic acid: chemical reconstruction of skin scars method. Dermatol Surg 2002;28(11):1017-21; discussion 1021.

23. Yug A, Lane JE, Howard MS, Kent DE. Histologic study of depressed acne scars treated with serial high-concentration (95%) trichloroacetic acid. Dermatol Surg 2006;32(8):985-90; discussion 990.

9

Salicylic Acid Peels

Niti Khunger

- Peel Formulations
- Equipment and Reagents
- Indications
- Contraindications
- Priming and Prepeel Preparation
- Procedure
- Postpeel Care
- Complications
- Bottomline

Introduction

Salicylic acid is a beta hydroxy acid (ortho-hydroxy benzoic acid), with a pKa of 3, commonly used as a peeling agent, either alone or in combination with other peeling agents. Unna, a German dermatologist, reported on the use of salicylic acid for chemical peels.[1] In the early 1990's, Swineheart reported satisfactory improvement of photoaging and pigmentary changes on the hands and forearms using 50% salicylic acid.[2] Salicylic acid is naturally present in certain plants and fruits and derived from sweet birch, willow bark and wintergreen leaves.

It is lipophilic and acts as a keratolytic agent by dissolving the intercellular lipids, surrounding the keratinized epithelial cells. Due to its lipophilic nature, it preferentially acts on the sebaceous follicle, has excellent comedolytic activity and hence is very useful for acne. It also has anti-inflammatory and antimicrobial properties. A derivative of salicylic acid, lipohydroxy acid has also been used in acne. It was found to be as efficacious.

Peel Formulations

It is available as salicylic acid powder, slightly soluble in water, but highly soluble in 95% ethanol, ether or methanol (common spirit). On application, the alcohol evaporates and the salt crystallizes on the skin forming a white precipitate. This appears like a frost and is called 'pseudofrost' because it is not true frosting which is seen with TCA due to coagulation of proteins.

- Hydroethanolic solution on a weight to volume basis. Salicylic acid powder 20 gm. Add 100 cc spirit or 95% ethanol to get 20%.
- Salicylic acid in a gel base is also available. The advantage of the gel is that no burning occurs on application. The disadvantage is that no pseudofrost is seen, hence uniform application of the peel cannot be judged. It has to be kept on the skin for a longer time as the peel penetrates slowly.
- A derivative of salicylic acid, capryloyl salicylic acid or beta-lipohydroxy acid (LHA) 5 to 10% has been used and found to be effective in lower concentrations. It showed slightly better results in a split—face study, when compared with glycolic acid for pigmentation and photoaging.[3]
- Salicylic acid paste (salicylic acid powder USP 50% methyl salicylate 16 drops, Aquaphor 112 gm). These can be used as body peels.

STORAGE

Store in glass bottles, away from light.

STABILITY

The concentration of the formulation of alcoholic solutions may increase due to evaporation of alcohol, when the bottle is repeatedly opened.

Equipment and Reagents

- Salicylic acid solutions 20%, 30%, 40%, 50%
- Alcohol to clean the skin
- Acetone to degrease the skin
- Cold water
- Petrolatum or Vaseline® to protect sensitive areas
- Syringes filled with normal saline for irrigation of eyes, in case of accidental spillage
- Glass cup or beaker in which the peeling agent is poured
- Cotton tipped applicators or swab sticks
- 2″ × 2″ cotton gauze pieces
- Gloves
- Head band or cap for the patient
- Fan for cooling.

Indications[4-8]

Salicylic acid peels are safe and can be used for all skin types I to VI.

- Acne
  - Comedonal acne
  - Inflammatory acne (Figures 9.1A to D)
  - Pigmented acne scars
  - Superficial acne scars (Figures 9.2A to C)
- Hyperpigmentation
  - Epidermal melasma (Figures 9.3A to D)
  - Postinflammatory hyperpigmentation

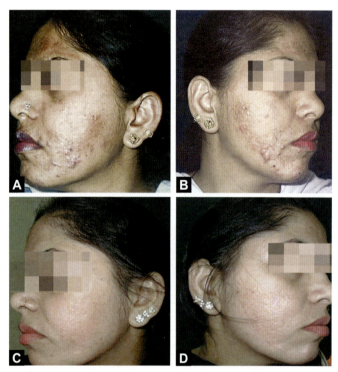

Figs 9.1A to D Active acne treated with 20% salicylic acid after 6 sessions at 2 weekly intervals along with systemic antibiotics. (A and B) Before treatment; (C and D) After treatment

- – Freckles
- – Lentigines.
- Photoaging
  - – Fine wrinkles
  - – Dyschromias.

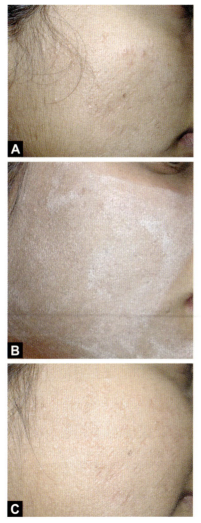

Figs 9.2A to C Superficial acne scars treated with 30% salicylic acid. (A) Before treatment; (B) Pseudofrost after application of 30% salicylic acid; (C) After 6 sessions every 2 weeks

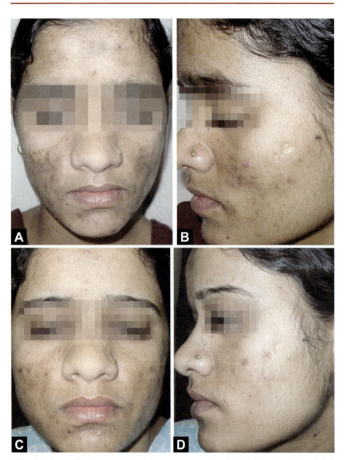

Figs 9.3A to D Acne with melasma treated with 20% salicylic acid, 6 sittings at monthly intervals. (A and B) Before treatment; (C and D) After treatment

- Textural changes
  - Oily skin
  - Rough uneven skin
  - Dilated pores.

- Keratotic lesions
  - Keratosis pilaris
  - Warts.
- Acne rosacea.

Contraindications

General contraindications include an allergy to salicylates or aspirin, pregnancy, lactation, unrealistic patient expectations and dermatitis at the peeling site.

Priming and Prepeel Preparation

As with all chemical peels, patient selection and counseling are important prerequisites to successful peeling. A detailed history and examination are essential. Detailed informed consent and photographic documentation are mandatory before peeling.

Priming and skin preparation vary according to the skin of the patient. In darker pigmented skins, priming should be done with hypopigmenting agents that are intended to be used postpeeling, such as hydroquinone, kojic acid, azelaic acid or arbutin. Patients should be repeatedly educated on the proper use of broad spectrum sunscreens and safe sun protection. Retinoids like tretinoin, adapalene or tazarotene should be used at night at least 2 to 6 weeks prior to peeling. They thin the stratum corneum, enhance epidermal turnover, decrease epidermal melanin, increase penetration of the peeling agent and expedite post-peel healing. Retinoid dermatitis, if any, must be controlled prior to peeling.

In patients with thin sensitive skins, retinoids should be stopped 1 week before the peel and resumed only after complete re-epithelialization.

Patients with photoaging benefit from 6 to 12% glycolic acid cream and retinoids as priming agents 2 to 4 weeks before peeling.

In patients with acne active infection should be controlled with systemic antibiotics before peeling. Azithromycin is preferable as both doxycycline and minocycline are photosensitizing.

Procedure

- The patient is asked to wash the face with soap and water.
- The hair is pulled back with a hairband or cap.
- The patient lies down with head elevated to 45° with eyes closed.
- Using 2″ × 2″ gauze pieces, the skin is cleaned with alcohol and then degreased with acetone or a prepeel cleanser which accompanies the kit.
- Sensitive areas of the face such as the lips, inner canthus of the eye and the nasolabial folds are protected with a thin layer of petrolatum.
- The initial peel should be done with 20% concentration to assess patient reactivity to the peel.
- Salicylic acid 20% is poured in a glass cup and quickly applied using a cotton-tipped applicator or a brush or a gauze piece. Application is done in a predetermined manner to the facial cosmetic units, starting from the forehead and progressing to the cheeks, chin, perioral area, nose and lower eyelids. The whole procedure should be completed within 30 seconds.
- Two to three coats are applied to get a uniform peel. Feathering strokes are applied at the edges, to blend with surrounding skin and prevent demarcation lines.
- The patient will experience a stinging and burning sensation which increases over the next 2 minutes, reaches a crescendo at 3 minutes and then rapidly decreases to baseline over the next minute. This is considered the end point of the peel. Some patients may experience mild anesthesia of the face due to the peel. Portable fans reduce the burning sensation.

- As the hydroethanolic vehicle evaporates, it leaves behind a white precipitate of salicylic acid on the surface of the face which is termed as salicylic acid frost or pseudofrost. This appears at about 30 seconds to 1 minute after applying the peeling agent. If there is an uneven area of salicylic acid frost the peel is reapplied in that area. The penetration of the active agent stops once the vehicle has volatilized. At this point there is no burning or stinging as the agent causes a superficial anesthesia to light touch. In a gel based peel no pseudofrosting is seen.
- The patient is instructed to wash the face with water and pat the face dry.
- A bland soapless cleanser like Cetaphil® may be used to remove traces of residual precipitate.
- Patients are then sent home with a moisturizer and instructed to limit sun exposure and use sunscreens appropriately.
- In case of salicylic acid gel peels, the peel is left over on the skin for 6 to 8 hours as the peel penetrates slowly.

Postpeel Care

Patients feel tightness of the skin after a peel. Sunscreens and moisturizers are used postpeel till desquamation subsides. Mild soap or nonsoap cleanser may be used. If there is crusting, topical antibacterial ointment should be used to prevent bacterial infection. They should avoid peeling or scratching the skin.

The topical skin regimen of hypopigmenting agents, acne medications, glycolic acid and retinoids is then resumed as appropriate, till the next peel. Peels can be repeated every 2 weeks, till satisfactory improvement. This usually occurs after 4 to 6 peels. Maintenance peels once a month or as and when required can be done thereafter.

Salicylic acid paste is used to treat dyschromias due to photoaging. It is applied under occlusion for 48 hours on the exposed areas of the neck, back and arms. Desquamation occurs that heals in 7 to 10 days.

Complications

The best way to avoid complications is to identify patients at risk and use lighter peels and good postpeel care. The patients at risk are those with a history of postinflammatory hyperpigmentation, keloid formation, and heavy occupational exposure to sun such as field workers, uncooperative patients and patients with a history of sensitive skin unable to tolerate sunscreens, retinoids and hydroquinone.

Complications are uncommon with salicylic acid peels and are usually mild and transient. Excessive crusting, desquamation, inflammation and erythema can occur (Figure 9.4). These should be treated aggressively to prevent PIH, particularly in skins of color. Frequent applications of moisturizers, topical steroid cream like hydrocortisone 1% are used to reduce side effects. More potent steroids are used if there is severe irritation. The skin returns to normal in 2 to 5 days. Bari et al. studied 268 patients with type IV and type V skin treated with 30% salicylic acid peels, weekly for various facial dermatoses such as acne and melasma and found it to be safe, with a low incidence of side effects.

Salicylism is not observed when applied on the face but has been reported when large amounts of 50% salicylic acid paste are applied to 50% of the body surface, under occlusion. It is characterized by tinnitus, dizziness, abdominal cramps and deafness. The patient should be asked to drink copious amounts of water to prevent salicylism.

Bottomline

ADVANTAGES

- Safe in all skin types I–VI

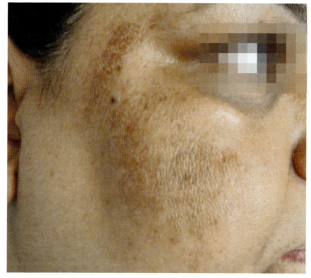

Fig. 9.4 Dryness followed by postinflammatory hyperpigmentation following 20% salicylic acid peel used for photoaging in type V skin

- Peeling action is self-limiting since it crystallizes within a short time on the skin surface
- Excellent peeling agent for acne
- Easy to visualize since it causes a white pseudofrost
- Causes superficial anesthesia
- Predictable results
- Less downtime.

DISADVANTAGES

- Limited depth of peeling, hence only superficial lesions can be treated.
- Causes burning when applied.

Conclusion

Salicylic acid peels are safe and well tolerated in all skin types, including skin of color. They give predictable results with less downtime. Salicylic acid is an excellent peeling agent for acne due to its lipophilic nature. It is effective for superficial epidermal conditions like epidermal melasma, oily skin, rough skin and mild photoaging. However, it is less effective in patients with significant photodamage due to limited penetration.

Key Points

√ Salicylic acid peels are safe for all skin types.
√ It is lipophilic and hence an excellent peeling agent for acne.
√ It has limited penetration and is effective for superficial epidermal conditions like oily, rough skin, epidermal melasma and mild photoaging.

References

1. Brody H. History of chemical peels. Chemical peeling and resurfacing, 2nd edn. St. Louis: Mosby Year Book Inc., 1997.pp.1-5.
2. Swineheart JM. Salicylic ointment peeling of the hands and forearms. J Dermatol Surg Oncol. 1992;18:495-8.
3. Oresajo C, Yatskayer M, Hansenne I. Clinical tolerance and efficacy of capryloyl salicylic acid peel compared to a glycolic acid peel in subjects with fine lines/wrinkles and hyperpigmented skin. J Cosmet Dermatol. 2008;7:259-62.
4. Vedamurthy M. Salicylic acid peels. Indian J Dermatol Venereol Leprol. 2004;70:136-8.
5. Grimes PE. The safety and efficacy of salicylic acid chemical peels in darker racial-ethnic groups. Dermatol Surg. 1999;25(1):18-22.
6. Lee HS, Kim IH. Salicylic acid peels for the treatment of acne vulgaris in Asian patients. Dermatol Surg. 2003;25(12):1196-9.
7. Ahn HH, Kim IH. Whitening effect of salicylic acid peels in Asian patients. Dermatol Surg. 2006;32(3):372-5; discussion 375.
8. Bari AU, Iqbal Z, Rahman SB. Tolerance and safety of superficial chemical peeling with salicylic acid in various facial dermatoses. Indian J Dermatol Venereol Leprol. 2005;71:87-90.

10

Tretinoin Peels

Niti Khunger

- Choosing a Peel Formulation
- Equipment and Reagents
- Indications
- Contraindications
- Priming and Prepeel Preparation
- Procedure
- Postpeel Care
- Complications
- Bottomline

Introduction

Retinoids are a class of polyisoprenoid lipids which include vitamin A (retinol) and its natural and synthetic analogs that play a role in epidermal cell regulation. They act by combining with retinoid receptors. Their role in the treatment of acne, hyperpigmentation and photoaging is well documented. Retinol and retinaldehyde are mild, less potent agents that are converted to retinoic acid. Tretinoin (transretinoic acid) and isotretinoin (13-cis-retinoic acid) are more active forms. Tretinoin is the most widely used topical agent. In lower concentrations (0.025%, 0.05% and 0.1%), it is used in acne, photoaging and priming the skin before peels and as maintenance therapy after peels. It has been used as a peeling agent in higher concentrations, 1 to 5%.[1-3]

Choosing a Peel Formulation

- Tretinoin peels 1 to 5% have been safely used for dark skins.
- Yellow peel contains salicylic acid, retinol, phytic acid, kojic acid, azelaic acid, vitamin C and bisabolol.

Equipment and Reagents

- Tretinoin solution 1%, 5% or yellow peel
- Alcohol to clean the skin
- Acetone to degrease the skin
- Cold water
- Petrolatum or Vaseline® to protect sensitive areas
- Syringes filled with normal saline for irrigation of eyes, in case of accidental spillage
- Glass cup or beaker in which the peeling agent is poured
- Cotton tipped applicators or swab sticks
- 2″ × 2″ cotton gauze pieces
- Gloves
- Head band or cap for the patient.

Indications

Tretinoin peels are safe and can be used for all skin types I–VI (Figures 10.1A to D).

- Acne
  - Comedonal acne
  - Inflammatory acne
  - Pigmented acne scars
  - Superficial acne scars
- Hyperpigmentation
  - Epidermal melasma
  - Postinflammatory hyperpigmentation
  - Freckles
  - Lentigines

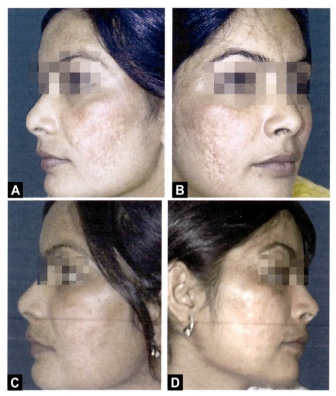

Figs 10.1A to D Acne with melasma treated with 1% tretinoin peel, weekly for 6 peels. (A and B) Before treatment; (C and D) After treatment

- Photoaging
  - Fine wrinkles
  - Dyschromias.

They have also been used for lightening of the underarms and to treat stretch marks.

Contraindications

They are contraindicated in patients with telangiectasia, blotchy erythematous ruddy complexion and rosacea, as they can increase vascularity. Other contraindications include pregnancy, lactation, unrealistic patient expectations and dermatitis at the peeling site.

Priming and Prepeel Preparation

Priming and skin preparations vary according to the skin of the patient. In darker pigmented skins, priming is done with hypopigmenting agents that are intended to be used post-peeling, such as hydroquinone 2 to 4%, kojic acid 2%, azelaic acid 10 to 20% or arbutin 5%. Patients should be repeatedly educated on the proper use of broad spectrum sunscreens and safe sun protection. Physical sunscreens containing zinc oxide or titanium dioxide are preferred. Retinoids like tretinoin, adapalene or tazarotene should be used at night at least 2 to 6 weeks prior to peeling. They thin the stratum corneum, enhance epidermal turnover, decrease epidermal melanin, increase penetration of the peeling agent and expedite post-peel healing. Retinoid dermatitis, if any, must be controlled prior to peeling.

In patients with thin sensitive skins retinoids should be stopped 1 week before the peel and resumed only after complete re-epithelialization.

Patients with photoaging benefit from 6 to 12% glycolic acid cream and retinoids as priming agents 2 to 4 weeks before peeling. In patients with active acne, infection must be controlled. Azithromycin is preferable as both doxycycline and minocycline are photosensitizing.

Procedure

After taking informed consent and photographs, the peel procedure is started.

- The patient is asked to wash the face with soap and water.
- The hair are pulled back with a hairband or cap.
- The patient lies down with head elevated to 45° with eyes closed.
- Using 2″ × 2″ gauze pieces, the skin is cleaned with alcohol and then degreased with acetone.
- Sensitive areas of the face such as the lips, inner canthus of the eye and the nasolabial folds are protected with a thin layer of petrolatum.
- Tretinoin 1% is poured in a glass cup and quickly applied using a cotton-tipped applicator or a brush or a gauze piece. Application is done in a predetermined manner to the facial cosmetic units, starting from the forehead and progressing to the cheeks, chin, perioral area, nose and lower eyelids. The whole procedure should be completed within 30 seconds.
- Two to three coats are applied to get a uniform peel. A uniform yellow frost is seen (Figure 10.2). The agent is reapplied in areas of irregular frosting. Feathering strokes are applied at the edges, to blend with surrounding skin and prevent demarcation lines.
- The advantage of tretinoin peel is that there is no burning sensation.
- The peel is left on for 4 hours and then the face is washed.

In a study of 15 patients with photoaging, 1 to 5% tretinoin peels were performed twice a week for five sessions.[1] Clinically, improvement was observed in the skin texture and appearance. On histopathologic examination, a decrease in the stratum corneum and an increase in the epidermal thickness were observed . In another study by Khunger et al. of 10 patients, skin type IV–V with melasma, 1% tretinoin peels were compared with glycolic acid 70% in a split face trial.[2] It was observed that a significant decrease in pigmentation occurred on both sides at 12 weeks ($p < 0.001$). There was no statistically significant difference between tretinoin and glycolic acid. Side effects were minimal and 1% tretinoin peel appeared to be well tolerated.

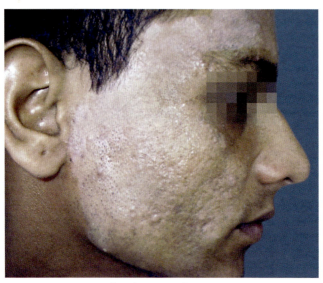

Fig. 10.2 Yellow frosting with 1% tretinoin peel

The yellow peel is a mild superficial peel and can be combined with other peels, like a low strength glycolic acid peel to increase efficacy. The 20% glycolic acid peel is first for 1 to 3 minutes till there is a faint erythema. It is neutralized followed by the application of the yellow peel. For a mild very superficial peel for brightening the skin and a glow a single layer is sufficient and left on for 4 to 6 hours. Two layers can be applied if the patient has thick oily skin. For a deeper peel, 3 to 4 layers are applied till there is a faint erythema.

Retinoic acid 5% peel has also been combined with microdermabrasion for enhanced results.[4] In a study of 6 patients with photoaging, 3 patients were subjected to microdermabrasion followed by retinoic acid 5%, while 3 patients applied retinoic acid 5% only. In both groups there was improvement in the texture, pigmentation, and appearance of the treated skin, clinically as well as on histology.

Postpeel Care

Patients feel tightness of the skin after a peel. Sunscreens and moisturizers are used postpeel till desquamation subsides. Mild soap or nonsoap cleanser may be used. The skin slowly peels without any discomfort in 2 to 3 days. Patients should avoid peeling or scratching the skin. With the yellow peel, desquamation occurs after 2 to 3 days and lasts for 3 to 4 days. Noncomedogenic moisturizers and sunscreen should be used, till the skin becomes normal.

The topical skin regimen of hypopigmenting agents, acne medications, glycolic acid and retinoids is then resumed as appropriate, till the next peel. Peels can be repeated till satisfactory improvement. This usually occurs after 4 to 6 peels. The tretinoin peels can be repeated every week and the yellow peel once a month.

Complications

Complications are uncommon with tretinoin peels and are usually mild and transient. Excessive desquamation, inflammation and erythema can occur. These should be treated aggressively to prevent postinflammatory hyperpigmentation (PIH), particularly in skins of color. Frequent application of moisturizers, topical steroid cream like hydrocortisone 1% are used to reduce side effects. More potent steroids are used if there is severe irritation. The skin returns to normal in 2 to 5 days. If PIH occurs, it should be treated with 5% hydroquinone and potent steroids.

Bottomline

ADVANTAGES

- Safe in all skin types I–VI
- Excellent peeling agent for acne, photoaging and melasma

- Easy to visualize since it forms a distinct yellow frost
- Causes no burning or discomfort
- Predictable results
- Less downtime.

DISADVANTAGES

- Limited depth of peeling, hence only superficial lesions can be treated
- Yellow color remains for 4 to 8 hours.

Conclusion

Tretinoin peels are safe and well tolerated in all skin types, including skin of color. They are excellent peeling agents for acne, photoaging and hyperpigmentation, without causing much inflammation or discomfort. They are effective for superficial epidermal conditions like epidermal melasma, oily skin, rough skin and mild photoaging. However, they are less effective in patients with significant photodamage due to limited penetration of the peeling agent.

Key Points

√ Safe in all skin types.
√ Excellent peeling agent for acne and mild photoaging.
√ Causes a yellow frost and has a limited depth of penetration of peeling.

References

1. Cucé LC, Bertino MCM, Scattone L, et al. Tretinoin peeling. Dermatol Surg. 2001;27(1):12-4.
2. Khunger N, Sarkar R, Jain RK. Tretinoin peels versus glycolic acid peels in the treatment of melasma in dark skinned patients. Dermatol Surg. 2004;30(5):756-60.

3. Kligman DE. Tretinoin peels versus glycolic acid peels. Dermatol Surg. 2004;30(12 Pt 2):1609.
4. Hexsel D, Mazzuco R, Dal'Forno T, et al. Microdermabrasion followed by a 5% retinoid acid chemical peel vs a 5% retinoid acid chemical peel for the treatment of photoaging—a pilot study. J Cosmet Dermatol. 2005;4:2:111-6.

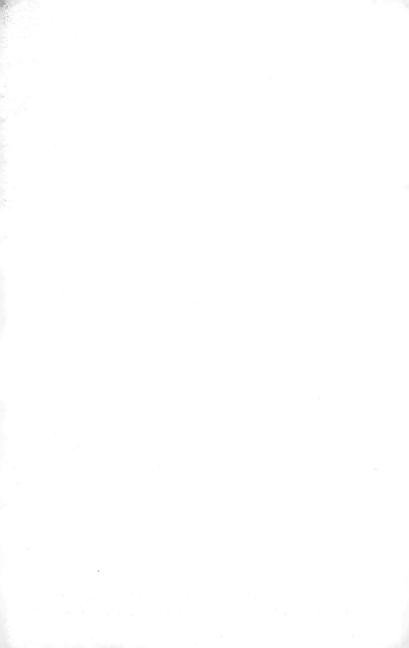

11

Jessner's Peel

Maya Vedamurthy, Amar Vedamurthy

- Mechanism of Action
- Choosing a Peel Formulation
- Equipment and Reagents
- Indications
- Contraindications
- Priming and Prepeel Preparation
- Procedure
- Postpeel Care
- Complications
- Combination Peels
- Bottomline

Introduction

Jessner's peel was popularized by Max Jessner as a superficial chemical peel. It is a combination of an alpha-hydroxy acid-lactic acid with a beta-hydroxy acid-salicylic acid, along with a phenol derivative—resorcinol. It is used alone or in combination with other peeling agents like trichloroacetic acid, to increase the depth of the peel. There have been subsequent modifications, where resorcinol has been replaced by citric acid, called modified Jessner's peel. Jessner's peel is not widely used in India, though it is an effective peeling agent.

Mechanism of Action

Jessner's peel is a combination of resorcinol, salicylic and lactic acid and therefore these molecules act in synergy. Resorcinol is a good peeling agent resulting in renewed stratum corneum and increased density of glycosaminoglycans. Lactic acid is an alpha hydroxy acid and salicylic acid is a lipophilic agent with keratolytic and anti-inflammatory properties.

Choosing a Peel Formulation (Table 11.1)

Table 11.1: Types of Jessner's peels			
Jessner's peel (Combe's peel)		*Modified Jessner's peel*	
Lactic acid	14%	Lactic acid	17%
Salicylic acid	14 gm	Salicylic acid	17 gm
Resorcinol	14 gm	Citric acid	8%
Ethanol to make 100 mL		Ethanol to make 100 mL	

Modified Jessner's peel eliminates resorcinol, reducing side effects and decreasing toxicity, while increasing efficacy.[1]

STABILITY

Jessner's solution is a light amber colored solution, with smell of resorcinol admixed with alcohol. Salicylic acid is light sensitive. Lactic acid is deliquescent and absorbs moisture; hence old crystals should not be used. Resorcinol should be used fresh as it turns dark on exposure to light and air. It usually has a shelf life of 2 years.

STORAGE

The solution has to be stored in a dark amber colored bottle with a tight cap. Do not expose to air.

Equipment and Reagents

- Correctly labeled reagent
- Alcohol to clean the skin

- Acetone to degrease the skin
- Cold water
- Syringes filled with normal saline for irrigation of the eyes, in case of accidental spillage
- Glass cup or beaker in which the required agent is poured
- Head band or cap for the patient
- Gloves
- Cotton tipped applicators or swab sticks
- 2″ × 2″ cotton gauze pieces
- Fan for cooling.

Indications

- Acne (Figures 11.1A and B)
- Actinically damaged skin

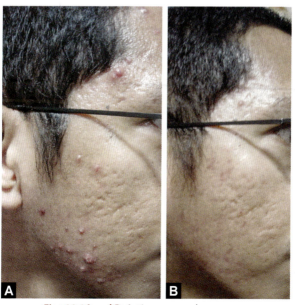

Figs 11.1A and B Active acne and acne scars treated with Jessner's peel

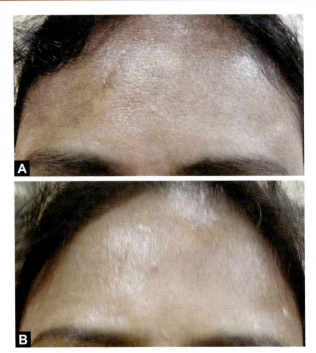

Figs 11.2A and B Melasma treated with Jessner's peel

- Dyschromias (Figures 11.2A and B)
- Superficial scars
- Dilated pores
- Fine wrinkles
- Keratosis pilaris.

Contraindications

ABSOLUTE

- Allergy to resorcinol

- Allergy to salicylates
- Pregnancy and lactation.

- Active infection
- Acne excoriée or obsessive picker.

Priming and Prepeel Preparation

Priming may or may not be done as it is a superficial peel and aggressive priming may inadvertently create a deeper peel than desired. However, in case of dyschromias priming with bleaching agent is essential. In thick oily skins, priming with retinoic acid, alpha-hydroxy acid or combination of both may be done. Before applying the peel, thorough cleaning to remove make up, oil and debris using alcohol, acetone or chlorhexidine is done. The aim is to degrease the skin and not to strip off any remaining stratum corneum.[2]

Procedure

- A test patch may be done behind the ear to assess allergies to resorcinol or salicylic acid. The solution is applied behind the ear over an area of 4 cm[2] and left on for 15 minutes. The test site is examined 4 days later for any allergic reaction.[3] An allergic reaction can manifest as pruritus, erythema and disproportionate edema.
- Jessner's solution is usually applied with a sable brush, but can also be applied with cotton-tipped applicators, gauze squares or cotton balls. The aim is to apply a uniform layer of acid to the entire treatment area. The application begins from the forehead, then the cheeks and then the face, chin and nose.
- The effect of Jessner's peel can be modified by the application of successive coats. Increasing the number of coats,

increases injury and depth of penetration. Rubbing the solution into the skin with a gauze square also enhances penetration. Three distinct levels of peels can be obtained.

- *Level 1:* This is achieved with a single coat. There is faint erythema followed by a light powder-looking whitening on the skin surface, which can be wiped off with a finger or wet cotton ball. This is a very superficial peel and will create only 1 to 2 days of mild flaking or no flaking at all.

- *Level 2:* It takes 2 or 3 coats to achieve this level. As the penetration of Jessner's solution is more, erythema becomes pronounced and turns bright red, rather than pink. Sometimes, there may also be few areas of true frosting. At this point patient feels a mild to moderate amount of burning and stinging, which lasts for 15 to 30 minutes, but may last for few hours. During the next two days, there is a persistent brownish red discoloration, which exfoliates for 2 to 4 days. The patient should be warned about the discoloration.

- *Level 3:* It is achieved with 3 or 4 coats. The skin shows prominent erythema with a significant number of pinpoint areas of frost, giving rise to a notable whitish look. Patients feel a moderate amount of stinging with this level of peel. During the next 2 days, there is a deeper brownish red discoloration followed by exfoliation, which lasts longer for 8 to 10 days. However no crusting or weeping is seen as this is only an intraepidermal peel.

- There can be variation in the level of peel and number of coats required, depending on the priming agent used, thickness of stratum corneum, sensitivity of the skin and the method of application. It takes 4 to 6 minutes for the full skin reaction to occur after each coat. Therefore, there should be an interval of 4 to 6 minutes between the coats and additional coats of the solution should not be applied until you have assessed how deep a peel you have already created.

- When applying over larger areas such as the arms, the patient is asked to drink a glass of water between the application of the coats and additional 4 glasses of water during the day.
- No neutralization is needed. Ice cold compresses may be given after washing the face with cold water.

Postpeel Care

Desquamation begins in the perioral area and then progresses across the face. If there is erythema or persistent stinging a mild topical steroid may be given 2 to 3 times a day. For dry flaky skin an emollient along with a sunscreen is recommended.

Complications

Complications are rare as Jessner's peels are superficial peels. Allergic reactions may occur to resorcinol or salicylic acid. Allergy to resorcinol can manifest as pruritic, erythema and disproportionate edema, 5 to 7 days after a peel.

In addition both resorcinol and salicylic acid have the potential to create systemic toxicity when used over large areas. Hence, caution should be used to avoid percutaneous absorption. Reactivation of viruses or secondary infection may occur, with deeper peels. Persistent erythema may pose a problem in few individuals. However, it can be successfully managed with mild steroid creams and bland emollients along with photoprotection.[4]

Combination Peels

Jessner's solution may be combined with trichloroacetic acid (TCA) to produce a combination chemical peel.[3] Usually, a single coat of Jessner's solution is applied and observed for a light frost. Next TCA 10 to 15% solution is applied evenly using a cotton tipped applicator. Individual areas may be retreated to achieve a deeper penetration for an actinic keratosis or deeper wrinkle. After a desired frost, cold saline compresses or ice pack is applied to make the patient comfortable. This combination peel is useful for treating photodamaged skin, pigmentary disturbances and fine wrinkles. Retinoic acid peels may also be combined with the above to achieve better results.

Bottomline

ADVANTAGES

- Safe peeling agent
- Gives rise to a lot of peeling that creates satisfaction in some patients.

DISADVANTAGES

- Toxicity can occur due to resorcinol or salicylic acid, if applied over large areas
- Causes a lot of stinging and burning
- There can be variation of manufacturing formulations
- Creates a lot of exfoliation that is not acceptable to many.

Conclusion

Jessner's peel is a useful peel for patients who want to "peel" and yet have only a superficial peel. It is a very safe peel as it is difficult to even in advertently create deeper wounds. It creates a fairly uniform depth peel, unlike alpha-hydroxy acids (AHAs). It is a useful agent in treating dyschromias.

Key Points

√ Jessner's peel is a safe peel.
√ It causes a lot of burning, stinging and exfoliation.
√ Useful for acne, photoaging and dyschromias.

References

1. Savant SS. Superficial and medium depth chemical peeling. In: Savant SS (Ed). Textbook of Dermatosurgery and Cosmetology. 2nd edn. ASCAD, Mumbai, India. 2005.pp.177-95.
2. Rubin MG. Jessner's peels. In: Rubin MG (Ed). Manual of Chemical Peels-superfical and Medium Depth. Ist edn. Philadelphia. JB Lippincot Co. 1995.pp.79-88.
3. Coleman WP III, Brody HJ. Combination chemical peels. In: Roenigk H, Roenigk R (Eds). Roenigk and Roenigk's Dermatologic Surgery, Principles and Practice, 2nd edn. Marcel Dekker Inc. New York. 1996.pp.1137-45.
4. Fulton JE Jr. Jessner's peel: In: Rubin MG (Ed). Chemical Peels. Procedures in Cosmetic Dermatology. Elsevier Inc. 2006.pp.57-71.

12

Newer Peels

Niti Khunger

- Mandelic Acid Peels
- Lactic Acid Peels
- Pyruvic Acid Peels
- Polyhydroxy Acid Peels
- Phytic Acid Peels
- Citric Acid Peels

Introduction

There has been a resurgence in the use of chemical peels to refresh and rejuvenate the skin and a variety of peels are being introduced for home care as well as for professional use. The aim of a chemical peel is to make the skin smoother with an even tone and texture and remove pigmentary dyschromias. The newer peels being introduced are gentler, with lower concentrations, available singly as well as in combinations. Many have added antioxidants and humectants to make them potent, with improved tolerance and less irritant potential.

Mandelic Acid Peels[1]

Mandelic acid (German mandel—almond) is an α-hydroxy acid, which can be obtained from amygdalin, a glycoside found in bitter almonds, peaches and apricots. The molecule of mandelic acid is larger than the glycolic acid molecule, hence penetration is slower. For chemical peeling 30%, 40% and 50% mandelic acid is used. Studies have shown improvement in photoaged skin, acne, abnormal pigmentation, and skin texture. It was found to be safe in darker skin types. It is the recommended AHA for those with sensitive skin since it is the least irritating. Though it has been used widely as a peeling agent, for acne, pigmentation and photoaging, either alone or in combination, there is a paucity of published scientific studies.

MECHANISM OF ACTION

The mechanism of action is similar to α-hydroxy acids. It causes dissolution of intercellular cement substance, stimulates collagen synthesis and promotes cellular regeneration. Mandelic acid has also been used in medicine for many years as a urinary antiseptic, known to inhibit *Staphylococcus aureus, Bacillus proteus, Escherichia coli*, and *Aerobacter aerogenes*. Chemically, mandelic acid has a structure similar to that of other well-known antibiotics. It is nontoxic and excreted in urine, after oral ingestion.

CHOOSING A PEEL FORMULATION

Mandelic acid has a pKa of 3.41 and is stronger than glycolic acid, which has a pKa of 3.83 at 25°C. It must be remembered that the acidity of AHAs may vary considerably with changes in temperature. Mandelic acid is partially soluble in water and freely soluble in isopropyl and ethyl alcohol. It is used in a concentration of 20%, 40% and 50% as a peeling agent. Lower concentrations of 2% are used as a facewash and 2 to 10% for home use.

Stability: Mandelic acid is stable and not light sensitive.

Storage: It should be stored in a cool place.

PROCEDURE

After usual skin preparation for a chemical peel, the agent is applied over the treatment area. It may be rubbed gently into the skin. Application time varies from 5 minutes to even longer. A personal open study of the use of mandelic acid 40%, in skin types IV–V was carried out for the treatment of resistant melasma and acne in 20 patients. Most of the patients experienced no burning or irritation and the application time was extended to 12 hours. Peels were repeated every 2 weeks for 6 peels. Eight out of ten patients with melasma (80%) and 9 out of 10 patients with acne (90%) improved, without any adverse effects.

BOTTOMLINE

Advantages

Mandelic acid has dual properties. It has antiaging properties similar to glycolic acid; hence it is useful for rejuvenating the skin and improving skin texture. It also has antibacterial properties; hence it is useful for acne (Figures 12.1A to D) and preventing gram-negative bacterial infections after laser-resurfacing. It is also effective for melasma and postinflammatory hyperpigmentation[2] (Figures 12.2A and B). Though mandelic acid is a stronger acid as compared to glycolic acid, its larger molecular weight, slows the penetration, making it less irritant. It is useful for patients with sensitive skin, infected acne and darker skin types. When compared with glycolic acid peels, then mandelic acid is less likely to result in crusting, blistering or other adverse effects on the epidermis. A notable difference between glycolic acid and mandelic acid products is the lack of skin irritation, erythema and burning that often accompanies skin treatments with glycolic acid preparations used for peeling.

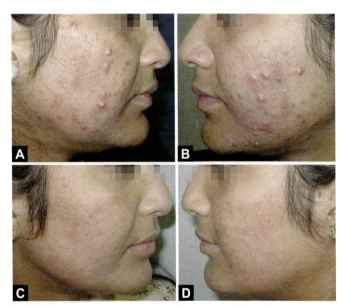

Figs 12.1A to D Acne treated with mandelic acid peels, 4 peels every 2 weeks

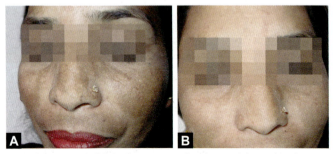

Figs 12.2A and B Melasma treated with mandelic acid peels, 8 peels every 2 weeks

Disadvantages

Since there is no irritation, burning or erythema, particularly in darker skins, it is difficult to pinpoint the endpoint of the peel. There is no obvious peeling, due to which there is lack of patient satisfaction, as to whether, the peel is actually working.

CONCLUSION

Mandelic acid is a promising peeling agent for the treatment of acne, melasma and photoaging in all skin types. The lack of irritation, burning and erythema are advantages over glycolic acid, making it an excellent lunchtime peel. However, long-term controlled scientific studies are needed to establish its efficacy as a peeling agent.

Lactic Acid Peels[2,3]

Lactic acid is an α-hydroxy acid, naturally occurring in sour milk, yogurt and tomato juice. It has one of the largest molecules among AHAs, so penetration is much slower which results in less irritation to the skin. It is a popular peeling agent for dry, sensitive skins as well as for lunchtime procedures as it causes virtually no peeling. As compared to glycolic acid, it is more hydrating and least irritating.

The mechanism of action of lactic acid is similar to glycolic acid as with all AHAs.

Their main action is to facilitate dissociation of the epidermal cells, leading to an increased desquamation of the stratum corneum and an increased regeneration. There is also an increase in the skin's content of natural hyaluronic acid that has water-holding capacity, which explains the moisturizing effect of AHAs. Due to these effects, the epidermis is somewhat thinned, smoother, with improved texture and scaling is reduced. The overall effect is skin which looks and feels smoother and better. It is a good peel to give a glow to the skin. AHAs can also reverse photodamage and reduce wrinkles, brown spots and roughness of the skin.

CHOOSING A PEEL FORMULATION

The formulation of lactic acid is critical for its use as a peeling agent. The pH or pKa is the determinant factor for all acids. Even a high concentration of acid at neutral pH is ineffective as less free acid is available. Lactic acid above a pH of 3.5 is used in cosmetics as a moisturizer. At a lower pH less than 3.5 in high concentrations lactic acid acts as a peeling agent. It is also a component of Jessner's peels along with salicyclic acid and resorcinol. It has also been used in combination with other peeling agents in varying concentrations (e.g. 10% lactic acid, 10% citric acid, 5% kojic acid, 2% hydroquinone, 2% salicylic acid, Percos India). Lactic acid is used as a 15 to 50% solution for home use applied weekly. Lactic acid 30% (pH 2.3) is used on sensitive, dry, oily, acne prone, or dehydrated skin. It is the weakest peel working gradually. A 40% solution (pH 2.2) is used on dry, dehydrated, and normal skin and is perfect for first time peel users. Lactic acid 50% (pH 2.0) is used for wrinkles and mature skin, as well as all skin types. Pure lactic acid full strength (92%, pH 3.5) is used as a peeling agent for professional use. Sharquie et al. reported lactic acid as a useful peeling agent for frictional dermal melanosis or Lifa disease.[4,5]

PROCEDURE

The procedure of application of lactic acid peels is similar to other peels. In a study of 30 patients with melasma, skin type IV, lactic acid 92% pH 3.5 was compared with Jessner's solution, applied every 3 weeks in a right left comparison study. It was found to be as effective as Jessner's solution.[3]

BOTTOMLINE

Advantages

Lactic acid has one of the largest molecular weight among AHAs, so penetration is much slower which results in less irritation to the skin. It can be safely used in patients with sensitive skin and patients with rosacea. Since lactic acid is a humectant it can also be used in patients with dry mature skin. It is also safer to start peeling with lactic acid in patients new to peels. Lactic acid acts as an exfoliator and moisturizer, removing the outer layers of thickened damaged skin and providing a smoother and healthier looking appearance. It also penetrates the deeper layers stimulating new collagen formation. It has also been useful in improving the barrier function of the skin. Since, it is naturally occurring in the skin, allergic reactions are extremely rare. With prolonged use, lactic acid has been found to be beneficial in improving dry skin, treating age related pigmentary dyschromias, improving oily and acne prone skin and decreasing fine lines and wrinkles.

Disadvantages

Lactic acid is a mild peeling agent and the improvement is gradual. Burning and irritation can sometimes occur. It can, however be combined with other peeling agents to hasten response.

CONCLUSION

Lactic acid has been well studied as a moisturizing agent, but less used singly as a peeling agent. It is more often utilized in combination with other peeling agents to counter dryness.

Pyruvic Acid Peels[6-8]

Pyruvic acid is an α-keto acid, recently formulated in a hydroethanolic vehicle at concentration of 40 to 70% for use as a superficial to medium depth peeling agent for the treatment of several dermatological diseases, including acne, post-acne scars, actinic keratoses, photoaging and warts. It is a potent acid due to its low pKa of 2.39 and small molecule allowing deeper penetration. It is physiologically converted partly to lactic acid and is a potent peeling agent.

Pyruvic acid induces detachment of keratinocytes, with thinning of the epidermis. It also penetrates into the papillary dermis causing dermoepidermal separation and stimulates production of collagen, elastic fibres and glycoproteins. It has also demonstrated antimicrobial and sebostatic properties.

CHOOSING A PEEL FORMULATION

The effect of pyruvic acid depends on the concentration used and the duration of application. Lower concentrations ranging between 40 to 50% are used as superficial peeling agents in a well-balanced proportion between water and ethanol and 70% is used for the treatment of warts. Pyruvic acid is also available in a gel form formulated with stabilized pyruvic and lactic acids. 25% pyruvic acid and 25% lactic acid are indicated for dark and sensitive skin; 40% pyruvic acid and 5% lactic acid, are indicated for acne, seborrhea and melasma; and 50% pyruvic acid and 5% lactic acid, treat photoaging, wrinkles, melasma and pigmentations (Percos, India) (Figures 12.3A and B).

PROCEDURE

After prepeel preparation, cleansing and degreasing the skin, the desired concentration of pyruvic acid is applied as cosmetic units on the face. It causes intense burning and stinging that is reduced with a fan. The peel is applied with a gauze and gently scrubbed, till erythema appears. It is then neutralized with 10% sodium bicarbonate in water solution. Treatment can be repeated every 2 to 4 weeks till improvement. In patients with warts and seborrheic keratosis, 70% solution is applied

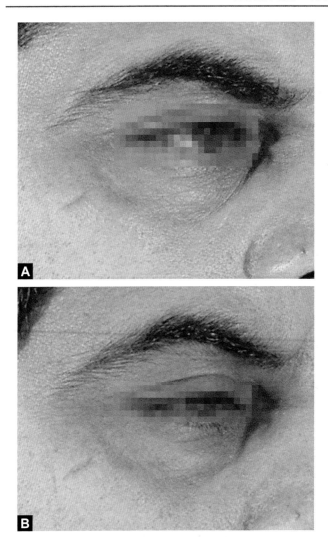

Figs 12.3A and B Dark undereye circles and aging improved after 4 pyruvic acid peels. (*Photo Courtesy* Dr VK Upadhyay)

as a paint twice a day for 2 to 3 weeks, depending on the size of the lesion. A study of 30 patients with papulopustular acne, with type IV–V skin, showed an average of 73.7% reduction in global acne scoring, with reduction in inflammatory and noninflammatory lesions.[8] Fifteen patients with melasma also showed a good response with a mean reduction of 3.5 in the Melasma Area and Severity Index (MASI) score.[8] In a study of 20 patients with mild photoaging, skin type II–III, pyruvic acid 50% showed a smoother texture, with reduction in fine lines and pigmentation.[6]

BOTTOMLINE

Advantages

Pyruvic acid is an α-keto acid that is less hydrophilic than α-hydroxy-acids because the –C=O group has a lower affinity for water molecules than the –OH group of α-hydroxy acids. Thus, pyruvic acid is well suited for treating oily skin and also has a strong comedolytic effect because of its lipophilic nature (Figures 12.3A and B). Postpeel erythema lasts only for 15 minutes and desquamation is very slight. Thus it is well tolerated.

Disadvantages

Pyruvic acid has been considered as a potent peeling agent and can penetrate up to the dermis causing deeper peels. Hence, it has a potential for scarring and should be used with caution over thin skin such as the eyelids.

CONCLUSION

Pyruvic acid has shown good results in inflammatory and noninflammatory acne, melasma and photoaging and is well tolerated in darker skins. However, it is a potent acid and should be used with caution.

Polyhydroxy Acids Peels[9-11]

Polyhydroxy acids are new generation of AHAs, similar in their action to AHAs but without the irritant reactions. They are potent antioxidants and also humectants and moisturizers. They have been found suitable for sensitive skin, including rosacea and atopic dermatitis. Polyhydroxy acids, including lactobionic acid and gluconolactone are often combined with other products and procedures to enhance efficacy.

Polyhydroxy acids are chemically and functionally similar to α-hydroxy acids. The significant difference is that the polyhydroxy acid has a larger molecular structure, which causes slower penetration, resulting in a reduction of irritation. Polyhydroxy acids used in skincare products are gluconolactone and lactobionic acid. Due to their multiple hydroxy groups (hence the name polyhydroxy acids), they attract and bind water and have humectant and moisturizing properties.

PROCEDURE

Lactobionic acids are potent antioxidants and improve barrier function of the skin. They are useful for sensitive skin and in the elderly as they are more moisturizing as compared to AHAs. Five peels with lactobionic acid peel at monthly intervals showed improvement in photoaged skin.[8] PHAs are often used before and after procedures such as laser therapy.

BOTTOMLINE

Advantages

Polyhydroxy acids do not cause stinging and burning. They are absorbed slowly, hence can be used on sensitive skin. They have in addition moisturizing properties, hence are useful in dry and mature skin. PHAs also act as antioxidants, hence have good antiaging properties. They are not photosensitizing, but reduce photoaging.

Disadvantages

Polyhydroxy acids are mild-peeling agents and hence, are generally used in homecare products. They can be used as peeling agents in combination with AHAs for sensitive skin.

CONCLUSION

PHAs like gluconolactone and lactobionic acid are mild-peeling agents that are useful in sensitive, dry and mature skin. They do not cause irritation, stinging and burning as compared to AHAs. They also have moisturizing, antioxidant and exfoliant properties, hence are useful for photoaging.

Phytic Acid Peels[12]

Phytic acid is an α-hydroxy acid with a large molecular weight. It is found naturally in cereals such as rice and wheat bran. It is a mild superficial peel that is safe for all skin types. It also has antioxidant properties.

PROCEDURE

This is a slow-release, mild superficial peel designed for those who either do not want or cannot afford to have a visible flaking of the skin. It contains a combination of α-hydroxy acids (AHAs) and phytic acid which is a strong antioxidant. Easy Phytic® evens out the complexion and has a marked tightening effect. It can help erase acne marks. The peel is applied and left over for 18 to 24 hours, before being washed away. This peel can be performed up to twice per week to achieve the desired results.

BOTTOMLINE

Advantages

It does not require neutralization. It is a slow superficial peel, hence can be safely used in all skin types.

Disadvantages

Since it is a superficial peel, it is useful only for mild epidermal conditions such as superficial hyperpigmentation, and for smoothening the skin. It requires multiple applications to have the desired results.

CONCLUSION

A phytic acid peel is a slow superficial peel that can be used safely in all skin types. It is also useful for sensitive skin. It does not require neutralization and can be kept on the skin for 18 to 24 hours. It needs to be repeatedly weekly for maximum results.

Citric Acid Peels[13]

Citric acid is a tricarboxylic acid with one hydroxyl group at the α position to one carboxyl group; at the same time the hydroxyl group is also at the beta position to the two remaining carboxyl groups. Therefore citric acid may be called an α-hydroxy acid or a beta hydroxy acid, depending on which carboxyl group is referred to. Citric acid is present as a carbohydrate metabolite in the skin. It is a powerful antioxidant.

Citric acid can produce an improvement of enlarged pores, freckles, lentigines, melasma and fine lines and wrinkles. It has been found that solutions containing citric acid are more effective at reducing the signs of photoaging than an equal concentration of glycolic acid at the same pH. In addition, side effects are less from citric acid as compared to glycolic acid. Lower concentrations of citric acid can be left on the skin without any adverse sequelae and are being used as peeling agents for home use.

PROCEDURE

Citric acid is used in a concentration of 10 to 50% as a home peeling agent and 20 to 70% as an office procedure. The skin is wiped with an alcohol, then degreased with acetone. The solution is left in place from approximately 2 to 5 minutes or until the patient develops a minor pink appearance to the skin. Then it is neutralized using a sodium bicarbonate solution, which produces bubbles. Once the bubbles have resolved the peel procedure is over. Alternatively, a water rinse can be used to neutralize the peel.

MISCELLANEOUS PEELING AGENTS

Tartaric acid is an α-hydroxy that is a dicarboxylic acid with two hydroxyl groups at the α positions of the acid, similar to the compound formed from two molecules of glycolic acid. Tartaric acid is nontoxic and occurs as a carbohydrate metabolite in the skin.

Malic acid is a dicarboxylic acid with one hydroxyl group at the α position of the acid, similar to the compound formed from one molecule of glycolic acid and one molecule of acetic acid. Malic acid is nontoxic and is present as a carbohydrate metabolite in the skin. These are all used in combination with other peeling agents.

Conclusion

Though there has been a lot of publicity in the media of these newer peels, there is not much published scientific evidence in peer reviewed journals of their efficacy and safety. Newer techniques are also being utilized, such as combination, segmental and sequential peeling to allow for increased benefit with fewer side effects. Thanks to rapid advances in chemical peel technology, these treatments can peel the skin, and actively treat the skin condition, with fewer side effects. If acne or pore size is the issue, components such as lactic acid, tretinoin, mandelic acid and resorcinol can be added. If there is hyperpigmentation, phytic acid, kojic acid, citric acid, mandelic acid and hydroquinone are useful. For sensitive skins, there are now chemical peels that use mild botanicals and soothing emollients, along with the key ingredients like lactic acid, phytic acid in order to treat the skin more gently. Therefore, chemical peels can now be personalized to benefit unique skin conditions and concerns.

Another advantage of the newer chemical peels is that they require very little downtime. After a chemical peel, often only mildly pink skin is seen that fades within a few hours. Later, the skin may or may not peel; hence peeling is no longer a requirement for the chemical peel treatment to be effective. A series of chemical peels is recommended in order to maximize results. Thus chemical peeling has become a powerful yet versatile tool for rejuvenating the skin.

Key Points

√ The newer peels like mandelic acid, lactic acid are safer for darker and sensitive skin.
√ They are mild peels that can be left over on the skin and do not cause obvious peeling thus having no downtime level.

References

1. Taylor MB. Summary of mandelic acid for the improvement of skin conditions. Cosmet Dermatol. 1999;12:28.
2. Taylor MB, Yanaki JS, Draper DO, Shurtz JC, Coglianese M. Successful short-term and long-term treatment of melasma and postinflammatory hyperpigmentation using vitamin C with a full-face iontophoresis mask and a mandelic/malic acid skin care regimen. J Drugs Dermatol. 2013;12:45-50.
3. Smith WP. Epidermal and dermal effects of topical lactic acid. J Am Acad Dermatol. 1996;35:388.
4. Sharquie KE, Al-Tikreety MM, Al-Mashhadani SA. Lactic acid chemical peels as a new therapeutic modality in melasma in comparison to Jessner's solution chemical peels. Dermatol Surg. 2006;32(12):1429-36.

5. Sharquie KE, Al-Dhalimi MA, Noaimi AA, Al-Sultany HA. Lactic Acid as a new therapeutic peeling agent in the treatment of lifa disease (frictional dermal melanosis). Indian J Dermatol. 2012; 57(6):444-8.

6. Ghersetich I, Brazzini M, Peris K, et al. Pyruvic acid peels for the treatment of photoaging. Dermatol Surg. 2004;30:32-6.

7. Griffin TD, Van Scott EJ, Maddin S. The use of pyruvic acid as a chemical peeling agent. J Dermatol Surg Oncol. 1989;15:1316-20.

8. Tosson Z, Attwa E, Al-Mokadem S. Pyruvic acid as a new therapeutic peeling agent in acne, melasma and warts. Egyptian Dermatology Online Journal. 2006;2(2):7.

9. Zoe Diana Draelos, Barbara A Green, Brenda L Edison. An evaluation of a polyhydroxy acid skin care regimen in combination with azelaic acid 15% gel in rosacea patients. Journal of Cosmetic Dermatology. 2006;5(1):23-9.

10. Grimes PE, Green BA, Wildnauer RH, Edison BL. The use of poly-hydroxy acids (PHAs) in photoaged skin. 02, Cutis. 2004;73(Suppl 2):3-13.

11. Bernstein, et al. Polyhydroxy acids (PHAs): Clinical uses for the next generation of hydroxy acids. Skin Aging. 2001;9(Suppl 9):4-11.

12. Deprez P. Easy phytic solution: A new α hydroxy acid peel with slow release and without neutralization. Int J of Cosmetic Surgery and Aesthetic Dermatology. 2003;5(1):45-51.

13. Bernstein, et al. Citric acid increases viable epidermal thickness and glycosaminoglycan content of sun-damaged skin. J Dermatol Surg. 1997;23:689-94.

13

Phenol Peels

Niti Khunger

- Mechanism of Action
- Choosing a Peel Formulation
- Equipment and Reagents
- Indications
- Contraindications
- Priming and Prepeel Preparation
- Procedure
- Phenol Application without Taping
- Postpeel Care
- Complications

Introduction[1]

Phenol as a peeling agent was described way back in 1882 by Unna, a German dermatologist and subsequently by Mackee in 1903. Various formulas were used but the most popular was the Gordon-Baker formula described in 1961. Traditionally, these phenol peels are used as deep peels and are contraindicated in darker skin types IV–VI due to the risk of permanent hypopigmentation. There have been recent modifications of phenol peeling formulas by Hetter[2,3] and Stone[4] and these modified phenol peels are now being used in darker skin types.

Mechanism of Action[5]

Phenol or carbolic acid is bactericidal and a local anesthetic in addition to its toxic effect. It acts as a protoplasmatic poison and causes enzyme inactivation, protein denaturation and increases permeability of the cell membrane leading to cell death. It penetrates deep into the reticular dermis and hence acts as a deep peeling agent. Aqueous liquefied 88% phenol in water, unoccluded, however, acts as a medium peel. In contrast to other agents, increasing the concentration of phenol actually decreases the penetration because the destruction forms a barrier to further penetration. When phenol is absorbed systemically through percutaneous application, it has a toxic effect on the cardiac, renal and hepatic tissues.

Choosing a Peel Formulation

Phenol is a weak acid with a pKa of 9.9, soluble in ethanol and ether and partially soluble in water.

BAKER-GORDON FORMULA[2]

Phenol, USP 88%	3 mL
Tap or distilled water	2 mL
Septisol liquid soap	8 drops
Croton oil	3 drops

Croton oil is an epidermal vesicant and increases penetration of phenol. This formula is not used in darker skin types.

STONE VENNER-KELLSON FORMULA

Liquefied phenol USP 88% (62.5% final phenol concentration)	60 mL
Septisol	10 mL
Distilled water	8 mL
Olive oil	5 mL
Croton oil (0.16%)	3 drops

STONE II FORMULA

Liquefied phenol USP 88%	
(60% final phenol concentration)	159 mL
Water	73.5 mL
Glycerin	4.5 mL
Croton oil (0.2%)	12 drops
Olive oil	3 drops

LITTON FORMULA

Phenol crystals 450 gm liquefied in 8 mL of distilled water and 8 mL of glycerin. 118 mL of liquefied phenol and 1 mL of croton oil followed by addition of 118 mL of distilled water is added.

Exoderm® Solution

Phenol liquid 91%	1 cc
Phenol crystalized 99%	1 cc
Distilled water	0.5 cc
Mixture of alcohol, olive oil,	
glycerine oil, and sesame oil	0.5 cc
Resorcin	0.3 cc
Citric acid	0.2 cc
Croton oil	2 drops
Soap	10 drops
Buffer tris	

Each component is essential for achieving optimal results and maximal safety. The chemical wounding agents are liquid phenol, crystallized phenol, resorcinol, and salicylic acid. The oils are croton oil, olive oil, glycerine oil, and sesame oil. The adjuvant components are distilled water, liquid hexachlorophene (septisol), ethanol (ethyl alcohol) and buffer tris solution.

Equipment and Reagents

- Phenol solution
- Alcohol to clean the skin
- Acetone to degrease the skin

- Spray of cold water
- Petrolatum or Vaseline® to protect sensitive areas
- Syringes filled with normal saline for irrigation of eyes, in case of accidental spillage
- Glass cup or beaker in which the peeling agent is poured
- Cotton tipped applicators or swab sticks
- $2'' \times 2''$ cotton gauze pieces
- Gloves
- Head band or cap for the patient
- Fan for cooling
- Equipment for cardiac monitoring
- IV fluids
- Sedating agents
- Phenol peeling requires an OT setup and presence of an anesthetist.

Indications

In darker skin type III–IV, with extreme caution:[5-10]
- Mild to moderate dyschromias
- Mild wrinkles
- Post acne scars.

In skin type I–II:
- Photoageing level III and IV
- Moderate to severe wrinkles
- Moderate to severe post acne scars
- Adjunct to other aesthetic procedures such as blepharoplasty.

Contraindications

- Cardiac disease
- Renal disease
- Hepatic disease
- Active bacterial, viral infection in the area to be peeled
- Active herpes simplex

- Open wounds, inflammation or irritation
- History of taking photosensitive drugs
- Uncooperative patient, e.g. patient is careless about sun exposure or application of medicine as directed
- Patient with unrealistic expectations
- History of abnormal scarring such as hypertrophic scars and keloids. Examine old scars and be cautious in patients with family history of keloids
- Atrophic skin or recent facial surgical procedures, within the last 6 months such as resurfacing, grafts, flaps etc. which may have compromised circulation and delayed healing
- Immunocompromised patients with delayed healing
- Isotretinoin use in the last six months
- Dark skin patients type V–VI.

Priming and Prepeel Preparation

Antivirals, valacyclovir 1 gm or famciclovir 500 mg tds is started on the day of the procedure and continued for 7 to 14 days till healing is complete. Prednisolone 30 mg is also started on the day of the procedure and continued for 5 days, to reduce postpeel edema and inflammation.

A mild sedative like diazepam 5 mg or lorazepam 1 to 2 mg may be given in anxious patients, the night before and on the day of the peel.

All other treatments such as scrubs, microdermabrasion, depilatories, waxing, bleaching and hair removal lasers should be avoided 1 week prior to peeling. Topical retinoids should be stopped 5 to 7 days before the peel to avoid uneven peeling.

Informed consent and photographic documentation are important prerequisites. Contact lenses should be removed before the peel.

Procedure

- The patient is best admitted in a day care center with all monitoring facilities

- – The procedure requires preoperative sedation with an intravenous line and preoperative IV hydration. Usually a liter of fluid is given preoperatively and in addition, a liter of fluid is given during the procedure. This is helpful in decreasing the phenol concentration from the serum.
- A pulse oximeter is attached to monitor cardiac activity.
- The patient is asked to wash the face with soap and water to remove dust and grime
- The hair are pulled back with a hairband or cap
- The patient lies down with head elevated to 45° with eyes closed
- Using 2″ × 2″ gauze pieces, the skin is cleaned with alcohol and then degreased with acetone
- The face is divided into zones and peeling is completed in one zone before proceeding to the next. This procedure is carried out over 90 minutes to reduce absorption and toxicity of phenol.

Application of Exoderm® with taping. The Exoderm® solution is applied with a cotton applicator and rubbed onto the skin and into all rhytides and skin folds starting at the forehead 2 mm behind the hairline. The phenol solution is applied with a 2″ × 2″ gauze piece. Gradually the whole forehead is covered, progressing to other cosmetic units such as periorbital, cheeks, perioral, and nose.[6]

The most painful area is the eyelid. An almost dry applicator is used up to the margin of the eye lashes at both angles. The solution is applied in the direction opposite to that of the eyebrows. Special attention should be given to the crow's-foot wrinkles and the periorbital region. The solution is vigorously rubbed into the unfolded rhytid prior to application. To avoid distinct lines of demarcation the solution must be applied 1 mm beyond the vermilion. The lower margin of application should be the earlobes and 2 cm below the mandibular line.

- On application, a white blanching or frosting of the skin is seen. As soon as frosting is seen, the area is rubbed dry with a dry cotton pad.

- The frosting then disappears in a few minutes and is replaced by a red-grayish color of the skin. The skin becomes edematous with puffy eyelids and feels "leathery" on touching. The procedure is performed twice in all facial areas, except for the deep folds and rhytides, which are treated three to four times. The total amount of solution does not exceed 3 mL.
- Following the procedure, the skin is taped by an impermeable, hypoallergenic, zinc-oxide-based plastic tape which is applied in strips of 3 to 4 cm in length in an overlapping fashion. The lower margin is taped up to the osseous part of the mandibula; the area beyond remains untaped.
- The tape mask is easily removed after 18 to 24 hours, exposing an edematous and pink skin.
- Immediately the face is covered by bismuth subgalate powder, which acts as a protective antiseptic and regenerative mask and remains for a period of 7 days.
- On the eighth day, vaseline is applied to the rigid powder mask in order to soften and detach the mask from the newly formed skin.

Phenol Application without Taping

Using the Stone VK formula or Stone II formula, a 15 second application per zone is sufficient to treat dyschromias in darker skins. Occlusion is done with a bland ointment.

- Piamphongsant[9] on the other hand, applied a modified phenol-castor oil peel for one minute only in 30 patients of dermal melasma, followed by an antimelasma cream. Two patients cleared completely in one week, whereas all the other patients had partial improvement. Hyperpigmentation was observed in 5 cases and hypopigmentation in 1 patient. Scar formation or cardiac arrhythmia was not observed in any case.

Postpeel Care

After the procedure, the patient is advised to use water-based moisturizing creams 4 to 5 times a day and sunscreen creams with a sun protection factor (SPF) of 15 to 19. The erythema gradually resolves over 2 to 6 weeks in the majority of cases. During this period, makeup is encouraged for blending face and neck skin color. In cases of olive skin patients (Fitzpatrick skin type 3 or 4), the application of hypopigmenting cream is recommended for the prophylaxis of postinflammatory hyperpigmentation.

Park et al[6] treated 46 Asian patients with facial acne scars, wrinkles with a modified phenol peel. (Exoderm®). They observed that 89% of patients with wrinkles and 64% of patiets with acne scars showed more than 51% improvement. Postinflammatory hyperpigmentation (PIH) was seen in 74% of patients while persistent hypopigmentation was also observed.

Complications

- Hypopigmentation can be persistent and even lifelong
- Lines of demarcation
- Hyperpigmentation rarely in darker skin types
- Persistent erythema
- Reactivation of herpes simplex
- Cardiac arrhythmias—in a study of 181 patients, mean age 56 years (range, 30–77 years), treated with modified phenol peels (exoderm), 12 patients (6.6%) developed cardiac arrhythmia during the procedure. It was more common in patients with diabetes, hypertension, and depression.[7,8] In 4 patients the arrhythmia was self-limited and did not require any intervention, while in the other 8 patients, 100 mg of lidocaine was given intravenously to control the arrhythmia.

Conclusion

Traditional phenol peels are contraindicated in darker skin types III–VI because of a high incidence of side effects, particularly persistent hypopigmentation. Phenol peels have been modified to make them effective and safer in olive skins. Various formulations are available but Exoderm® and Stone VK formulae are more popular. They are now being gradually used in darker skins for the treatment of facial acne scars and rejuvenation of the face. However, reports in Indian patients are lacking. It would be worthwhile to see the results in dark skin patients, living in tropical climates, where there is prolonged sun exposure.

However, the main disadvantage of deep phenol peeling is that it requires an OT setup with facilities for anesthesia, presence of an anesthetist and carries a higher risk of cardiac complications. Though results with a single peel are rather dramatic, as compared to superficial and medium peels, the significant downtime involved, prolonged healing and higher risk of complications often deter patients and physicians alike from performing deep peels. The trend, nowadays, is towards, safer, gentler treatments with virtually no downtime.

Key Points

√ Phenol is a deep peeling agent requiring an OT setup and cardiac monitoring.
√ It can cause permanent hypopigmentation.
√ Traditional phenol peels are used only in type I and II skin types.
√ Modified phenol peels are being used in skin types III–IV.
√ It has a significant downtime.

References

1. Brody H. History of Chemical Peels. Chemical peeling and resurfacing, 2nd edn. St. Louis: Mosby Year Book Inc., 1997.pp.1-5.

2. Hetter GP. An examination of the phenol-croton oil peel: Part I. Dissecting the formula. Plast Reconstr Surg. 2000;105(1):227-39; discussion 249-51.

3. Hetter GP. An examination of the phenol-croton oil peel: Part II. The lay peelers and their croton oil formulas. Plast Reconstr Surg. 2000;105(1):240-8; discussion 249-51.

4. Stone PA. The use of modified phenol for chemical face peeling. Clin Plast Surg. 1998;25(1):21-44.

5. Yoon ES, Ahn DS. Report of phenol peel for Asians. Plast Reconstr Surg. 1999;103(1):207-14; discussion 215-7.

6. Park JH, Choi YD, Kim SW, et al. Effectiveness of modified phenol peel (exoderm) on facial wrinkles, acne scars and other skin problems of Asian patients. J Dermatol. 2007;34(1):17-24.

7. Landau M. Advances in deep chemical peels. Dermatol Nurs. 2005;17(6):438-41.

8. Landau M. Cardiac complications in deep chemical peels. Dermatol Surg. 2007;33(2):190-93; discussion 193.

9. Piamphongsant T. Phenol-castor oil: Modified peel for dermal melasma. Dermatol Surg. 2006;32(5):611-7; discussion 617.

10. Yoram Fintsi, Marina Landau. Exoderm: Phenol-based peeling in olive- and dark-skinned patients. Dermatol Surg. 2006;32(5):611-7; discussion 617.

14

Nonfacial Peels

Niti Khunger

- Difference between Facial and Nonfacial Peels
- Patient Assessment
- Indications
- Priming
- Procedure
- Postpeel Care
- Complications

Introduction

Photoaging involves not only the facial skin but also involves the neck, exposed areas of the chest, back and forearms. Treating only the face can lead to sharp areas of demarcation and mismatch between facial and nonfacial areas. Hence patients often seek treatment of nonfacial areas. Another common complaint, particularly in older women is macular amyloidosis seen on the upper back and upper arms. It is refractory to treatment and chemical peels may be an adjuvant therapy in selected cases. In addition, acne on the back, chest and upper arms often heals with pigmentation, especially in darker skins, that can persist for a long time. Postacne scarring is also common in darker skins, particularly in males. Though chemical peeling is not as popular on nonfacial areas as compared to facial peeling, it is an option in selected patients.

Difference between Facial and Nonfacial Peels[1,2]

- Traditionally, chemical peeling of nonfacial areas is considered to be risky due to increased incidence of complications. During the process of wound healing, regeneration of skin is from the pilosebaceous glands. The density of these glands is thirty times lower on the neck and trunk and approximately forty times lower on the dorsa of the arms and hands. Since nonfacial skin contains fewer appendages as compared to facial skin, re-epithelialization is delayed, leading to increased risk of complications.
- Postpeel care is difficult and often neglected in these areas, due to contact with clothing.
- Superficial peels are usually not very effective for nonfacial skin, while medium and deep peels can give rise to unpredictable results. Repeated superficial peels have to be carried out to achieve results. Deep peels are contraindicated in darker skins, due to risk of permanent pigmentary changes.
- Peeling agents have to be applied to larger areas; hence risk of systemic toxicity is more, especially with salicylic acid, resorcinol and phenol peels.
- The upper chest, back and arms are sites prone to developing scarring and keloid formation, hence deeper peels should be done cautiously.

Patient Assessment

Before peeling the patient, the following factors should be thoroughly assessed:
- Skin type
- Degree of photodamage
- Previous surgical treatment
- History of hypertrophic scaring, keloids, acne, allergies

- Current medications including isotretinoin, photosensitizing drugs
- Degree of sun exposure
- Patient expectations.

Indications

- Photoaging (Figures 14.1A and B)
- Postacne pigmentation and mild postacne scarring
- Postinflammatory hyperpigmentation (Figures 14.2A and B)
- Cutaneous macular amyloidosis (Figures 14.3A to C)
- Keratosis pilaris
- Striae distensae.

CONTRAINDICATIONS

- History of hypertrophic scars and keloid formation
- Diabetes
- Immunosuppression
- Previous radiation or surgery that can cause delayed healing.

Priming

Skin should be primed with sunscreen, retinoic acid, glycolic acid and hydroquinone at least 4 to 6 weeks before peeling. Tretinoin and glycolic acid should be stopped 1 week prior to the peel.

Procedure

Skin is cleansed with alcohol and degreased with acetone.

For superficial pigmentary dyschromias a superficial peel, repeated at monthly intervals is effective.

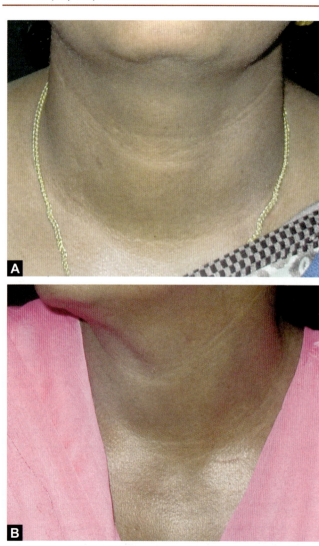

Figs 14.1A and B Combination of salicylic acid and glycolic acid peels for melanosis of the neck after 8 sittings at weekly intervals

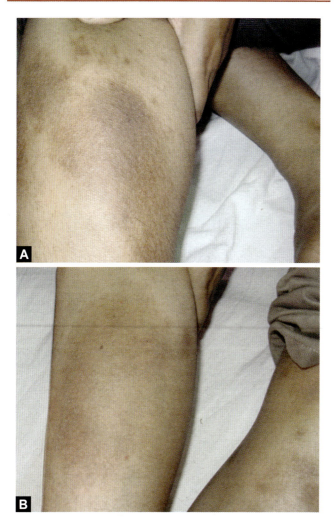

Figs 14.2A and B PIH following lichen planus on the legs treated with sequential peels. 50% salicylic acid, followed by glycolic acid hydroquinone peels. (Glyco K) at weekly intervals. (A) Before treatment; (B) After 2 sessions

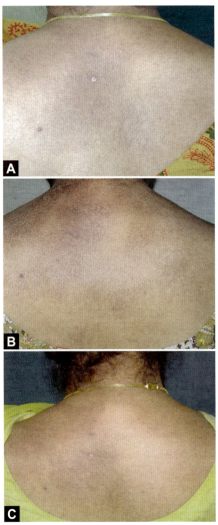

Figs 14.3A to C Sequential peel 50% salicylic acid followed by 15% TCA. (A) Before treatment; (B) After 1 month; (C) After 2 months

Peeling in nonfacial areas can be done with salicylic acid, glycolic acid or trichloroacetic acid (TCA). Salicylic acid used as a paste is applied.[2,3] Care must be taken not to apply over large areas to avoid salicylism. A hydroalcoholic solution can also be used in a concentration of 20 to 30%.

A medium depth peel is applied for significant photo-damage. Glycolic acid 70% in gel form followed immediately by TCA 40% has shown good results (Cooks peel).[4] Repeated applications of TCA are done till the endpoint is reached.

The endpoint is development of erythema with a speckled frost. In areas of greater photodamage, peeling can be deeper till light uniform frosting is seen. However, care should be taken in darker skins.

When the desired endpoint is reached, it is neutralized with large amounts of 10% sodium bicarbonate. For localized lesions, spot peels can be done. To prevent lines of demarcation, feathering at the edges with lower concentration of peeling agent can be carried out.

Chemical peels can cause temporary improvement in the appearance of keratosis pilaris. For keratosis pilaris, a combi-nation of a home regimen containing an exfoliating agent like salicylic acid, alpha hydroxy acid and tretinoin combined with chemical peeling with 70% glycolic acid can show significant benefit. These should be combined with skin lightening agents like hydroquinone to prevent postinflammatory hyperpigmen-tation (PIH) in dark skinned patients.

Striae distensae can also be treated with combination treat-ments with chemical peels. Subcision combined with chemical peeling or microneedling combined with chemical peeling can offer benefit in mature hypopigmented striae distensae on the trunk and flexural areas. TCA 15 to 20% or glycolic acid 35% may be used. Microneedling is done with a narrow eye roller 0.5 to 1.0 mm length.

Postpeel Care

Emollients are prescribed till the skin peels. Tretinoin and hydroquinone are restarted after one week. Scaling and flaking continue for 2 to 4 weeks and complete healing may take upto one month. It is essential to avoid sun exposure during this period. Peel may be repeated after one month, if desired.

Complications

Complications are similar to peeling in facial areas, except the risk of delayed healing, secondary infection, pigmentary alterations, textural changes and scarring are increased.

Conclusion

Nonfacial peels are indicated mainly for the treatment of photoaging, acne and acne scars, PIH and pigmentary dyschromias on the neck, chest, back and upper arms. Though healing takes approximately double the time in these areas as compared to the face, the risk of complications can be greatly reduced by taking proper precautions in the postpeel period. Alternative methods of treating photodamage in the nonfacial areas such as dermabrasion, CO_2 laser resurfacing also lead to complications. Er:YAG laser has been reported to be safer. However, in a study of the Er:YAG laser used for rejuvenation of the neck and hands, cosmetic improvement was only minimal in a majority of the patients and complications such as bacterial infection and hyperpigmentation were observed in a few patients.[5]

Repeated superficial peels at monthly intervals can be carried out safely in all skin types. Though medium peels are more effective, they should be performed cautiously in darker skins, as they can lead to persistent hyper or hypopigmentation and keloids.

Key Points

√ Nonfacial peels are mainly indicated for photoaging, dyschromias and postacne scars on the neck, upper chest and arms.
√ Healing time is prolonged due to fewer appendages in these areas, hence there is a higher risk of complications.
√ Repeated superficial monthly peels are safer than deeper peels.

References

1. Savant SS. Superficial and medium depth chemical peeling. In: Savant SS (Ed). Textbook of Dermatosurgery and Cosmetology, 2nd edn. ASCAD, 2005.pp.177-95.
2. Rubin MG. Salicylic acid peels (nonfacial). In: manual of chemical peels-superficial and medium depth, Ist edn. Philadelphia. JB Lippincot Co., 1995.pp.103-8.
3. Gladstone HB, Nguyen SL, Williams R, et al. Efficacy of hydroquinone cream (USP 4%) used alone or in combination with salicylic acid peels in improving photodamage on the neck and upper chest. Dermatol Surg. 2000;26(4):333-7.
4. Cook KK, Cook WR Jr. Chemical peel of nonfacial skin using glycolic acid gel augmented with TCA and neutralized based on visual staging. Dermatol Surg. 2000;26(11):994-9.
5. Jimenez G, Spencer JM. Erbium: YAG laser resurfacing of the hands, arms, and neck. Dermatol Surg. 1999;25(11):831-4; discussion 834-5.

15 Combination and Sequential Peels

Niti Khunger, Shenaz Arsiwala

- Combination Peels
- Sequential Peels
- Segmental Peels
- Switch Peels
- Complications
- Phytic Acid Peels

Introduction

The clinical effect of chemical peeling is removal of superficial skin lesions, regeneration of new tissue with improvement of the skin texture and long lasting therapeutic and cosmetic benefits. Various peeling agents are available, with differing mechanisms of action, making peeling a very versatile procedure for different skin types. The concept of combining different peeling agents was introduced in the seventies by Brody, when solid CO_2 was combined with TCA 35% in a series of 3000 patients.[1] Monheit[2,3] and Coleman[4] furthered this concept.

The requirements of the cosmetic units of the face often differ in the same patient. Application of the peeling agents can thus be customized according to various segments of the face using segmental peels. These mix and match options give chemical peeling a newer dimension for treating patients optimally, with minimal downtime and risks.

Combination Peels

Combination peels combine two or more different agents in a single formulation. The advantages of combination peels are multiple. The range of action of a single peel can be increased by combining agents that complement their actions. The depth and efficacy of the peel can be increased. It can also improve the safety of formulations as lower concentrations of individual agents are used. The earliest and most widely used combination peel is Jessner's solution. However, many of these combination peels are proprietary. They contain lower concentrations and are left over peels that can be safely used in darker skin types. Some peels are in gel formulations where the chemical agents are slowly released reducing side effects.

SUPERFICIAL PEELS

- *Jessner's solution:* Lactic acid 14 gm, salicylic acid 14 gm, resorcinol 14 gm with ethanol added to make 100 mL. (Can be remembered by the pnemonic LASER) (Figures 15.1A and B).
- *Modified Jessner's solution:* Lactic acid 17%, salicylic acid 17 gm, citric acid 8% with ethanol added to make 100 mL.
- Lactic acid 10%, citric acid 10%, kojic acid 5%, hydroquinone 2%, salicylic acid 2%. (Melaspeel KH Sesderma peels, Spain—Percos scientific, India). It is used for facial and neck pigmentation, photoaging and priming before laser therapy.
- Arginine 20%, lactic acid 15%, aloe vera 1%, allantoin 0.5% (Argipeel Sesderma peels, Spain—Percos scientific, India). Used for facial rejuvenation, decreasing fine wrinkles and pore size and under eye dark circles (Figures 15.2A and B).
- Combination of glycolic acid 33%, citric acid 10%, kojic acid 10%, lactic acid 9%, salicylic acid 5%, willow herb extract and bearberry extract (Glicopeel K Sesderma peels, Spain—Percos scientific, India) (Figures 15.3A to D).

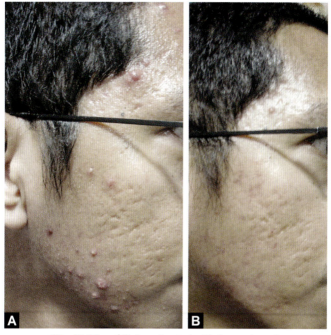

Figs 15.1A and B Acne treated with Jessner's peel
(*Photo courtesy:* Dr Maya Vedamurthy)

- Salicylic acid 20%, mandelic acid 10% in gel form (SM Peel, Timpac Engineers) (Figures 15.4A to D).
- Lactic acid 35% + glycolic acid 25%
- Mandelic acid 15% + Lactic acid 15%, a low strength peel for sensitive skin, mandelic acid 30% + lactic acid 40%. Chemical peels with mandelic acid combined with lactic acid, at weekly or bi-weekly intervals, have shown improvement for melasma, lentigenes, and fine photoaging. They are particularly useful for patients with sensitive skin.

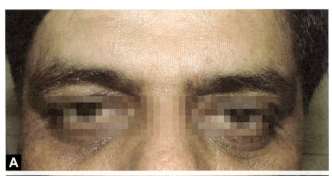

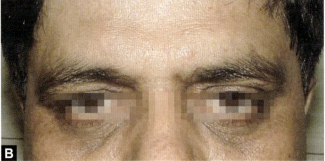

Figs 15.2A and B Arginine peel for under eye rejuvenation
(*Photo courtesy:* Dr VK Upadhyay)

- Retises-CT® has ampoules containing 10% ascorbyl 2-glucoside (vitamin C) along with sachets containing 15% lactic acid, 4% retinol and 1% retinaldehyde.
- Yellow peel facial contains the following active ingredients: salicylic acid, retinol, phytic acid, kojic acid, azelaic acid, vitamin C and bisabolol. This peel is reapplied two to three times every 20 to 30 minutes till the skin feels hot. For a superficial peel, reapplication is done three to four times till the appearance of erythema.

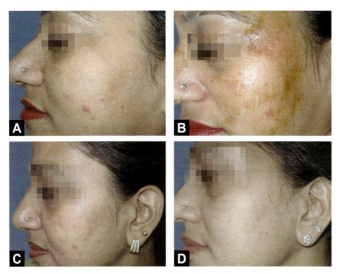

Figs 15.3A to D Glycolic kojic acid combination peel for melasma

- Slow release combination peel with phytic acid, glycolic acid, lactic acid and mandelic acid. (Easy phytic peel®)
- The fluor-hydroxy pulse peel is a combination of 5-fluoro-uracil 5% lotion and glycolic acid 70% (Drogaderma, Sao Paulo, Brazil). It has been successfully used for the treatment of actinic keratoses and disseminated actinic porokeratoses.[5,6]

The precise formula used may be adjusted to meet each patient's needs. For example, patients with oily thick skins and acne will benefit from higher concentrations of salicylic acid, while patients with predominant hyperpigmented lesions benefit from higher concentrations of hydroquinone, kojic acid and citric acid along with glycolic acid. Patients with sensitive skin can tolerate lactic acid and mandelic acid safely. In a personal study, 30 patients with resistant melasma with type

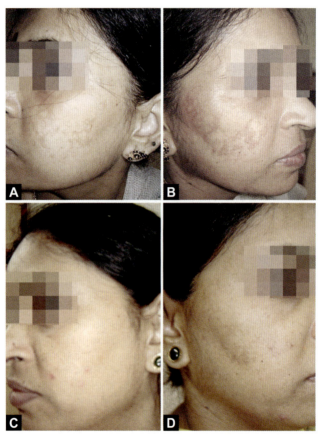

Figs 15.4A to D Salicylic-Mandelic acid peel for melasma
(*Photo courtesy:* Dr Vivek Mehta)

IV–V skin were treated with a combination peel of glycolic acid 33%, citric acid 10%, kojic acid 10%, lactic acid 9%, salicylic acid 5%, willow herb extract and bearberry extract (Glicopeel K Percos scientific, India). The peel was left on the skin for 12 hours, without any side effects. There was an improvement of 40 to 80% of melasma (average 70%) in all patients, when applied every 2 weeks for 12 applications. It has been observed that patients with dark skins do not tolerate resorcinol, hence resorcinol paste is not very popular. Jessner's solution has also been observed to cause PIH in V–VI skin types, hence should be used with precaution (personal observation).

Sequential Peels

Sequential peels are chemical peels using more than one peel at a time in a sequential manner as they may not be compatible in a single formulation. The need for the sequential peel arises from the fact that the pKa of different chemicals may not be similar hence the use of optimal strength of these chemicals in a single formulation may not be practicable. The advantage is that the peel that is applied first exfoliates the skin and enhances penetration of the second peel leading to a greater depth of the peel. These are medium depth peels and should be used with proper precautions and priming in dark skin patients. Priming with sunscreens and hypopigmenting agents should be done at least 2 to 4 weeks prior to sequential peels.

- Glycolic acid 70% combined with TCA 35% (Coleman's Peel).[3] The glycolic acid is applied first followed by the application of TCA. No prepeel defatting is necessary. Glycolic acid 70% is applied for 2 minutes, the solution is washed off and then TCA 35% is applied. This is a strong medium depth peel and should be avoided in darker skins.
- Modification: In dark skins prone to postinflammatory hyperpigmentation (PIH), the concentration of TCA should be lowered to 15 to 25%. In the nonfacial areas like the neck, back or arms, TCA concentration should be lowered to 15 to 20% and then gradually increased. For photoaging, hyperkeratotic lesions like seborrheic keratoses, dermatosis papulosa nigra and actinic keratoses are treated first with electrosurgery or radiofrequency and the peels are applied after healing.

- Jessner's solution with 35% TCA. (Monheit's peel).[2] The Jessner's solution is applied first followed by application of TCA. It is useful for pigmentation and photoaging but less successful for depressed scars.
- Salicylic acid 20 to 30% can be applied sequentially with glycolic acid 35%. First salicylic acid is applied, and then washed off after formation of pseudofrost followed by application of glycolic acid 35%. This leads to greater penetration of glycolic acid with reduced side effects due to lower concentrations. It is particularly useful for darker skins, where the chances of PIH are reduced.
- Salicylic acid 20 to 30% can also be applied sequentially with trichloroacetic acid. First salicylic acid is applied, then washed after formation of pseudofrost and cessation of burning. It is then followed by application of trichloroacetic acid 10 to 25%, depending on the site and thickness of the skin. This leads to greater penetration of trichloroacetic acid with reduced side effects due to lower concentrations. It is particularly useful for darker skins, where the chances of PIH are reduced (Figures 15.5A to D).

The advantage of sequential peels is that a greater depth of the peeling agent can be obtained without increasing concentration. Hence, they are useful for conditions that have a dermal component such as mixed melasma, lichenoid pigmentation and PIH.

Segmental Peels

Segmental peels consist of using different peels in different cosmetic units, at the same session. The choice of the peeling agent depends on the condition being treated, the severity in different cosmetic units and the type of patient's skin. For example, a patient with melasma and acne can be treated with a peel containing glycolic acid, hydroquinone and kojic acid on the cheek and comedones on the nose and forehead are treated with salicylic acid 20 to 30%.

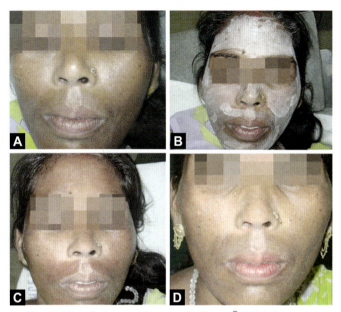

Figs 15.5A to D Sequential peel, salicylic acid® 20% followed by glycolic acid 70% after 2 weeks

The under eye area is treated with higher concentration of TCA in mature skins to reduce pigmentation and fine lines, while the cheeks and forehead can be treated with lactic acid or glycolic acid to improve pigmentation.

Switch Peels

The beauty of chemical peeling is that it is easily possible to switch from one peel to the other, tailoring the peeling agents according to the requirement of the patient, as the condition improves. When the peels are changed serially in different peeling sessions, they are called switch peels. It gives a greater flexibility in choosing a peeling protocol from patient to patient, hence leading to greater patient and professional satisfaction.

Complications

Complications can occur with any peel; however the incidence is reduced when combination peels are used. Medium depth peeling with TCA 50% can lead to scarring, whereas combining a lower concentration of TCA 35% (15–25% in skin type IV–VI) with glycolic acid or Jessner's solution leads to significant improvement with reduced incidence of scarring and pigmentary complications. It should be remembered that combining two peeling agents in a sequential manner can increase penetration of the second peeling agent and increase the depth of the peel, with increase risk of complications. Hence the concentration of the second peeling agent should be lowered, than what is normally used.

Phytic Acid Peels[7]

INTRODUCTION

Phytic acid is an alpha hydroxy acid with a large molecular weight. It causes a mild superficial peel that is safe for all skin types. It also has antioxidant properties.

The easy phytic peel works on the controlled release principle, where there is a slow progressive release of the constituents of the peel. This ensures complete penetration and full action of all components in the solution. Easy phytic peel is composed of 3AHAs, glycolic acid, lactic acid and mandelic acid with phytic acid. The 3 AHA's have different rates of penetration in the epidermis, with glycolic acid going in first, followed by lactic and mandelic acid, being less volatile goes in last. The release and action of each is progressive and hence this peel does not need to be 'neutralized' by the physician. Although the solution has a very low pH 0.5 to 1 lower than its pKa, it cannot cross the buffer potential of the skin and so self-neutralization occurs automatically in the skin. The acid penetration is complete and yet every molecule in the solution remains fully active.

MECHANISM OF ACTION

The acids work at the keratinocytes level, and they can move down to epidermis and progressively reach upper dermis without exceeding the skin's normal capacity to buffer the acids and gradually they lose the aggressiveness working to full capacity. Like any other AHA's they work by increasing the epidermal thickness, regulate keratinization, reduce intercorneocyte cohesion, enhance hydration, and improve quality of elastin and collagen. Mandelic acid has antibacterial and anti-inflammatory properties and is a helpful adjuvant in active acne. Mandelic acid is also known to improve hyperpigmentation and so helpful in acne with pigmented scars in Asian skins. The phytic acid in the easy phytic solution is a large inositol hexaphosphoric acid which fights and neutralizes free radicles. The peeling promotes cell regeneration but during this process it also releases damaging free radicles. Phytic acid reduces the cell degeneration induced by free radicles. Once the AHA's have made the skin permeable, the phytic acid penetration is faster inciting free radicle neutralization and reducing the inflammation in postpeel period.

INDICATIONS

- Acne, particularly with erythematous scars (Figures 15.6A to D)
- Photoaging
- Hyperpigmentation.

PROCEDURE

- *Priming:* All products acting on stratum corneum are prohibited in 2 to 3 weeks preceding easy phytic peels as

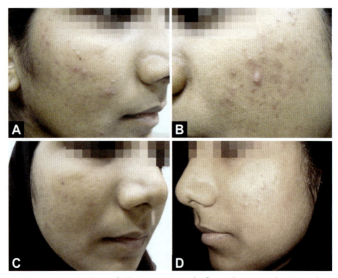

Figs 15.6A to D (A and B) Active acne before phytic peels; (C and D) Improvement in acne and acne scars after 2 phytic acid peels at weekly intervals). (*Photo courtesy:* Dr Shenaz Arsiwala)

these agents should penetrate the skin slowly. Any acids or exfoliants that erode the corneal layer allowing solution to penetrate quickly increases the risk of complications and diminishes the effect of slow release of the constituents. Sun protection is essential at all times as a standard peel protocol.

• A neutral pH cleanser is used to clean the skin. About 2 to 2.5 cc of the peeling solution is taken on cotton ball and applied gently and evenly. Coats can be repeated, but should not be rubbed. The patient will feel a tingling sensation which fades away. It should not be neutralized. A postpeel cream is applied when the tingling sensation fades away.

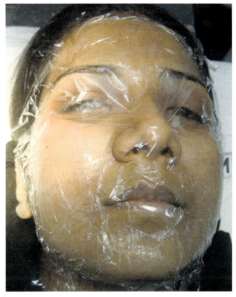

Fig. 15.7 Application of cling film. (*Photo courtesy:* Dr Shenaz Arsiwala)

- The face is then covered with a cling film (impermeable cellophane film) for 20 to 30 minutes and then removed. Post peel occlusion with cling film prevents evaporation of transepidermal water and water-soluble components, increases skin temperature locally and enhances penetration of cream applied (Figure 15.7).
- The cream is left on till next morning, and the patient should refrain from cleansing, scratching or rubbing the face till next morning. Regular sunscreen is started after normal cleansing in the morning.
- No frosting should appear and a strict vigilance is mandatory as for any other peels. In case of accidental frosting (this may happen if retinol or exfoliating agents have been used)

the peel becomes a standard AHA peel. In the postpeel period, swollen red dots indicate deep dermal penetration and dermal edema, which fades in 2 to 3 days. Sunscreens should be continued throughout the period of peeling.

- The peel can be repeated after 10 to 14 days.

Conclusion

Peeling agents can thus be combined in the form of combination peels, sequential peels and segmental peels to enhance efficacy, without increasing concentration, thus minimizing adverse effects. These mix and match options give chemical peeling a newer dimension for treating patients optimally, with greater versatility and satisfaction at the same time reducing risks.

Key Points

√ Chemical peeling agents can be used in various ways singly or in combination for maximum effect with minimum risk.
√ These options add a new dimension for treating patients optimally.

References

1. Brody HJ, Hailey CW. Medium depth chemical peeling of the skin: a variation of superficial chemosurgery. J Derm Surg Oncol. 1986;12:1268-75.
2. Monheit GD. The Jessner's + TCA peel: A medium-depth chemical peel. J Dermatol Surg Oncol. 1989;15:953-63.
3. Monheit GD. The Jessner's-trichloroacetic acid peel. An enhanced medium-depth chemical peel. Dermatol Clin. 1995;13(2):277-83. Review.
4. Coleman WP III, Futrell JM. The glycolic, trichloroacetic acid peel. J Dermatol Surg Oncol. 1994;20:76-80.
5. Marrero GM, Katz BE. The new fluor-hydroxy pulse peel. A combination of 5-fluorouracil and glycolic acid. Dermatol Surg. 1998; 24(9):973-78.

6. Teixeira SP, de Nascimento MM, Bagatin E, et al. The use of fluor-hydroxy pulse peel in actinic porokeratosis. Dermatol Surg. 2005; 31(9 Pt 1):1145-8.
7. Philippe Deprez. Easy phytic solution: A new alpha-ahydroxy acid peel with slow release and without neutralization. International Journal of Cosmetic Surgery and Aesthetic Dermatology 2003;5(1): 45-51.

16

Combination Therapies

Niti Khunger

- • Patient Counseling
- • Chemical Peel with Microdermabrasion
- • Chemical Peel with Dermasanding
- • Chemical Peel with Dermabrasion
- • Chemical Peel with Lasers
- • Chemical Peel with Botulinum Toxin
- • Chemical Peel with Fillers
- • Chemical Peel with Microneedling
- • Chemical Peel with Subcision
- • Complications

Introduction

Chemical peeling has been used as a time-tested procedure for resurfacing and rejuvenation of the skin. With the advent of alternative techniques such as dermabrasion, ablative lasers, microdermabrasion, nonablative lasers and light sources, the use of peels declined. However, lately there has been a resurgence in the use of peels, due to standardization of peels and peeling procedures, leading to safer peels, with fewer side effects and predictable results.

In addition, combining peels and different procedures has led to an increased efficacy, with a reduced risk of complications. Treatment can be tailored to individual needs at different cosmetic areas of the face, hence leading to less aggressive procedures and decreased healing times.

While planning combination procedures, it is essential to first analyze the skin type of the patient, the degree of aging and rejuvenation procedures required at different cosmetic areas.

Patient Counseling

As with any aesthetic procedure, an informed detailed pre-operative consultation is a prerequisite to patient satisfaction results. It is an optimal time to define patient's motivation for the desired cosmetic improvement, address the patient's fears and develop a plan of action in close coordination. It is important to have an expectation alignment with the patient. If need be repeated consultations are done, utilizing the intervening period for starting home care products and judging the ability of the patient to follow skin care as prescribed. Problematic patients with unrealistic expectations should not be taken up, particularly for invasive procedures. The expected degree of improvement, related risks and expected downtime should be discussed before initiating any interventional rejuvenation procedure.

Chemical Peel with Microdermabrasion[1,2]

Microdermabrasion is an aesthetic procedure for very super-ficial skin smoothening using aluminum oxide crystals. Few studies have reported on the combination of microderma-brasion combined with superficial chemical peeling to enhance outcomes. Microdermabrasion alone does provide the benefits of exfoliation but provides faster results and increased patient satisfaction when combined with superficial glycolic acid (alpha-hydroxy acid) peels because of the significant antiaging effects of glycolic acid peels. In one study , the combination of microdermabrasion followed by a 5% retinoic acid peel showed slightly greater improvement in the histological alterations resulting from photoaging as compared to peeling alone, though clinical differences were not significant.[1]

Chemical Peel with Dermasanding[3-5]

Dermasanding is a procedure where sterile sandpaper is used to abrade the skin, up to a level of the papillary dermis. This is followed by chemical peeling. The advantage is that a greater depth of peeling is possible, without increasing the concentration of the peeling agent. Secondly sandpaper abrasion is not very uniform and leaves minute islands of normal skin, hence re-epithelialization is quicker, with a reduced downtime. Since lower concentrations of peeling agents are used, pigmentary changes are less common and improve faster, particularly in darker skin types. This combination technique of dermasanding with chemical peel has been popular for the treatment of postacne scars. It has also been used for the treatment of stretch marks, a condition difficult to treat.

Adatto and Deprez[5] treated 69 female patients with stretch marks at various sites such as the abdomen, lateral thighs, breasts, back and wrist with sand abrasion followed by a patented peel solution Easy Peel® containing carboxylic acid, L-ascorbic acid, citric acid, excipients and 15% TCA.

This was followed by application of a patent peel under plastic occlusion for 6 to 24 hours. An improvement of 70% was seen after 1 to 8 treatment (median 4.2) in striae of all types fresh and old.

PROCEDURE (FIGURES 16.1 TO 16.9)

- Sterile sandpaper (medium grade P220, wet or dry) is cut into 2 × 8 cm strips. It is rolled around an empty 2 or 5 cc sterile syringe.
- After surgical cleansing, the area is marked with a surgical pen. For the treatment of depressed acne scars, the scars are marked, where deeper dermasanding would be required.

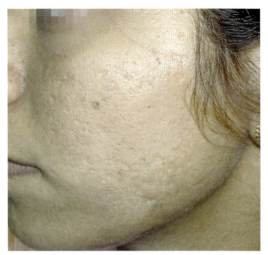

Fig. 16.1 Postacne scars

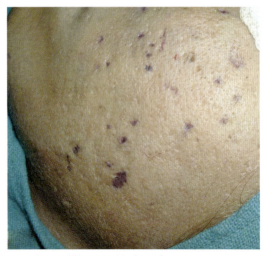

Fig. 16.2 Marking the scars

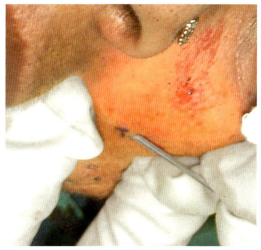

Fig. 16.3 Subcision

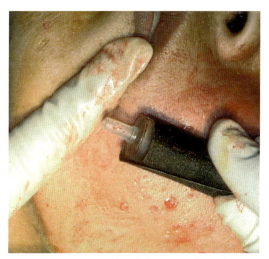

Fig. 16.4 Manual sand abrasion with sterile sandpaper rolled on a 2 cc syringe

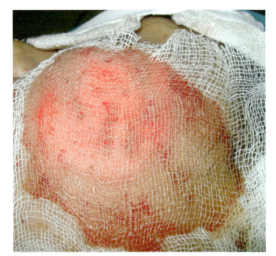

Fig. 16.5 Gauze piece soaked with 2% lignocaine and adrenaline

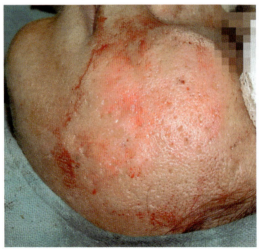

Fig. 16.6 Bleeding controlled

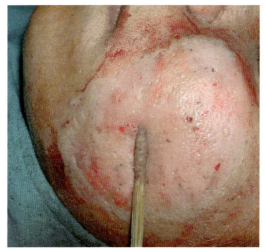

Fig. 16.7 Fifteen percent TCA applied

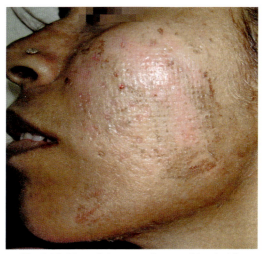

Fig. 16.8 Manual dermasanding combined with TCA 15%, postacne scars—after 1 week

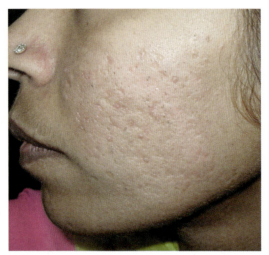

Fig. 16.9 Manual dermasanding combined with TCA 15%, postacne scars—after 3 weeks

- Skin is stretched and the rolled sandpaper is rubbed till pinpoint bleeding is seen. For the treatment of striae, there should be no bleeding, only discomfort.
- A single layer of gauze is put over the abraded area and it is moistened with 2% lignocaine with adrenaline. This reduces the bleeding and provides anesthesia after about 3 to 5 minutes.
- Chemical peeling is then done with 15% TCA till a uniform white frost is seen. Slight burning may occur.
- The area is then cleaned with normal saline and the edges are feathered with 10 to 15% TCA, to prevent demarcation lines.
- The wound is dressed with a nonadherent dressing, which is removed after 1 week.
- At 1 week there is mild erythema that resolves gradually. Sunscreens should be started postprocedure, when re-epithelialization is complete. Mild topical steroids, like

1% hydrocortisone (Cutisoft) or 1% desonide (Desowen) may be used if erythema is severe or persistent beyond two weeks. Hypopigmenting agents, which were used for priming are restarted after 2 weeks, to prevent post-inflammatory hyperpigmentation in darker skins.

- For deeper acne scars, after dermasanding the depressed punched out scars are elevated using a punch (punch elevation) and larger scars are excised and sutured (Figures 16.10 to 16.13).
- Complications that can occur are persistent erythema, hypopigmentation and hyperpigmentation, and lines of demarcation (Figure 16.12).
- The improvement is about 40 to 60% with this procedure. It has been observed that for postacne scars, results are better initially and the skin appears smooth, probably due to edema. Subsequently after 1 to 2 months there is a gradual reduction in improvement, as edema resolves. However,

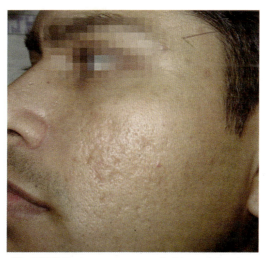

Fig. 16.10 Postacne scars treated with sand abrasion followed by chemical peel with 15% TCA

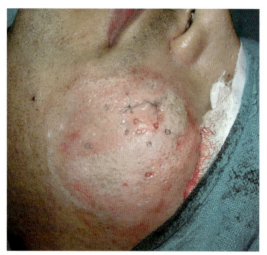

Fig. 16.11 Acne scars treated with sand abrasion, punch elevation, followed by chemical peeling with 15%, TCA

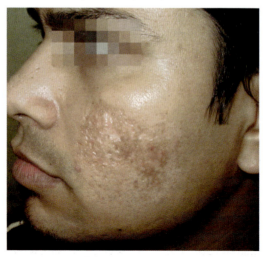

Fig. 16.12 Line of demarcation with hyperpigmentation

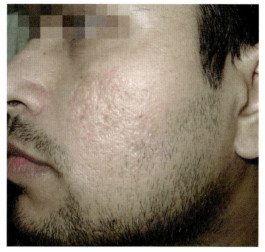

Fig. 16.13 Improvement after 1 month

the incidence of complications is much less as compared to medium depth and deep peels and dermabrasion (Personal observation).

Chemical Peel with Dermabrasion[6-8]

Chemical peeling can be combined with dermabrasion (chemabrasion). This procedure was originally used by combining application of 50% TCA followed by dermabrasion for postacne scarring. However, 50% TCA caused scarring and is now not advocated. In one study, focal chemical peeling was combined with carbon dioxide (CO_2) laser, scar excision, punch grafting, and dermabrasion for the treatment of acne scars.[8] Initially, focal chemical peeling was performed on all patients with TCA, followed by CO_2 laser, scar excision, and punch grafts for deep scars. Finally, dermabrasion was done for the remaining scars. Excellent or good results were observed in 75% of patients. The degree of improvement increased on follow-up and number of focal chemical peeling procedures.

Chemical Peel with Lasers[4,9]

Chemical peeling can also be combined with laser resurfacing for skin rejuvenation. First a chemical peel is performed and then the deeper wrinkles in the periorbital and perioral areas are treated with pulsed CO_2 laser. Chemical peels can also be combined with nonablative skin rejuvenation.

Chemical Peel with Botulinum Toxin[10]

Botulinum toxin can be used to relax muscles causing dynamic wrinkles on the forehead, frown lines, crows feet and perioral region. This is followed by chemical peeling. The advantage is that as new collagen is formed, there is minimal muscle movement, hence the remodeling is better. Results are immediate due to the toxin, while collagen deposition occurs over a period of 4 to 6 months.

Chemical Peel with Fillers[10]

Fillers can be used to increase volume and help in atrophic wrinkles and depressed scars. They have an additive effect as they affect the deeper portion, while chemical peeling affects the superficial signs of photoaging and texture. Superficial temporary fillers (Restylane®, Hylaform®, Esthelis®) are best used after chemical peeling, when inflammation subsides and complete healing occurs. Residual scars and wrinkles can be treated. Semipermanent and permanent fillers (fat, sculptra, radiesse) are better used 4 to 8 weeks prior to the resurfacing procedure.

Chemical Peel with Microneedling

Chemical peels can be safely combined with microneedling for acne scars. The advantage is that the chemical peel improves the surface texture and hyperpigmentation, whereas the microneedling improves the atrophic scars. The depth of the needles for microneedling should be varied according to the indication and area. For example, for facial rejuvenation, microneedles should be 0.5 to 1.0 mm in size, depending on thick or thin skin. For acne scars it should be 1 to 5 to 2.5 mm depth, depending on the severity of acne scars. In a comparative study, 35% glycolic acid peeling combined with microneedling gave superior results as compared to microneedling alone.[11]

Chemical Peel with Subcision

Chemical peeling can also be combined with subcision in the same session for treatment of acne scars. The subcision is performed first, followed by the chemical peel. For example, salicylic acid peel can be used to decrease pigmentation along with subcision.

Complications

Complications are more common when dermabrasion is combined with chemical peels as it can lead to greater penetration of the peeling agent with increased risk of scarring. The common complications that can occur when peels are combined with microdermabrasion or manual dermasanding are persistent erythema, hypopigmentation, hyperpigmentation, and lines of demarcation.

Conclusion

The approach to chemical peeling for facial rejuvenation has now expanded beyond a single-stage procedure. Chemical peels are an excellent addition to other esthetic procedures.

They can be used with ongoing home treatment with lower concentration of alpha hydroxy acids and retinoids. They can be combined optimally with other facial procedures such as ablative and nonablative lasers and light therapies, microdermabrasion, dermabrasion, botulinum toxin, fillers, blepharoplasty and face lifts. It is now frequently the combination of treatments that produces desired results in the shortest possible time, with minimal downtime. Each facial concern is customized and addressed individually with the appropriate modality. Chemical peels are here to stay and their recent re-emergence either alone or as combination procedures proves their efficacy in the treatment of medical and cosmetic disorders.

Key Points

√ Chemical peeling can be combined with different techniques to optimize results.
√ Surface irregularities like rough texture and hyperpigmentation are improved with chemical peels, while deeper scars and wrinkles are corrected with fillers and botulinum toxin.
√ Combining sandabrasion with light chemical peels is a popular technique for acne scars and striae.
√ Combining superficial chemical peels with nonablative rejuvenation modalities are promising technique.

References

1. Hexsel D, Mazzuco R, Forno TD, et al. Microdermabrasion followed by a 5% retinoid acid chemical peel vs. a 5% retinoid acid chemical peel for the treatment of photoaging—a pilot study. Journal of Cosmetic Dermatology. 2005;4:2:111-6.
2. Briden E, Jacobsen E, Johnson C. Combining superficial glycolic acid (alpha-hydroxy acid) peels with microdermabrasion to maximize treatment results and patient satisfaction. Cutis. 2007;79 (1 Suppl Combining):13-6.

3. Harris DR, Noodleman FR. Combining manual dermasanding with low strength trichloroacetic acid to improve actinically injured skin. J Dermatol Surg Oncol. 1994;20(7):436-42.

4. Fulton JE, Rahimi D, Helton P, Dahlberg K. Neck rejuvenation by combining Jessner/TCA peel, dermasanding, and CO_2 laser resurfacing. Dermatol Surg. 1999;25:745-50.

5. Adatto MA, Deprez P. Striae treated by a novel combination treatment—sandabrasion and a patent mixture containing 15% trichloroacetic acid followed by 6-24 hrs of a patent cream under plastic occlusion. J Cosmet Dermatol. 2003;2(2):61-7.

6. Stagnone JJ. Chemabrasion, a combined surgical technique of chemical peeling and dermabrasion. J Dermatol Surg Oncol. 1977;3:217-9.

7. Ayhan S, Baran CN, Yavuzer R, et al. Combined chemical peeling and dermabrasion for deep acne and post-traumatic scars as well as aging face. J Am Acad Dermatol. 1999;40(1):95-7.

8. Whang KK, Lee M. The principle of a three-staged operation in the surgery of acne scars. J Am Acad Dermatol. 1999;40:95-7.

9. Effron C, Briden ME, Green BA. Enhancing cosmetic outcomes by combining superficial glycolic acid (alpha-hydroxy acid) peels with nonablative lasers, intense pulsed light, and trichloroacetic acid peels. Cutis. 2007;79(1 Suppl Combining):4-8.

10. Landau M. Combination of chemical peelings with botulinum toxin injections and dermal fillers. Journal of Cosmetic Dermatology. 2006;5(2):121-6.

11. Sharad J. Combination of microneedling and glycolic acid peels for the treatment of acne scars in dark skin. J Cosmet Dermatol. 2011;10:317-23.

17

Chemical Peeling in Darker Skin

Niti Khunger

- Differences
- Problems
- Patient Assessment
- Counseling
- Priming and Preparation
- Precautions
- Peel Selection
- Procedure
- Postpeel Care
- Complications

Introduction

Skin color is one of the most striking variations in humans. In sunny climates, people tend to have darker and thicker skins. Melanin filters out UV light, protecting against sunburn and cutaneous malignancies. Apart from melanin, genetic, environmental and other unknown factors also play a role in variations of skin color. In the last few decades, increasing globalization has created multiracial countries leading to the formation of a wide range of different shades of skin colors and hair types among the world's population. Apart from pigmentation, darker skins are also qualitatively different, in terms of thickness and texture. Various terms are used to describe nonwhite skins such as 'ethnic skin,' 'skin of color,' 'darker skin', 'richly pigmented skin', etc.

Differences[1]

Although no quantitative differences in melanocytes are observed, the melanocytes in dark skin produce greater quantity of melanin with singly dispersed, heavily melanized melanosomes. Within the keratinocytes, the melanosomes contain more melanin and show a slower degradation. The most important difference that is clinically relevant is that melanocytes show hyper-reactivity to minor skin trauma, resulting in postinflammatory hyperpigmentation (PIH). Light-skinned individuals, on the other hand, display smaller melanosomes clustered in membrane-bound groups that appear to be broken down much more quickly within keratinocytes. Increased epidermal melanin provides greater photoprotection, hence photodamage, ageing, actinic keratoses, skin wrinkling and skin malignancies are relatively uncommon and these tend to occur later as compared to fair skins. However, dyschromias are much more common (Figures 17.1A and B).

Problems[2]

Dyschromic changes and postinflammatory reactions of hyper or hypopigmentation appear to be more common and more noticeable in patients with increased skin pigmentation. Melanocytes show labile and exaggerated responses to cutaneous injury. In the case of postinflammatory hyperpigmentation, excessive melanin synthesis and/or abnormal distribution of melanin occurs. A variety of chemical mediators of inflammation and cytokines may be involved. The excess melanin may then be transferred into keratinocytes (epidermal hyperpigmentation) or moved into the dermis to persist within macrophages (dermal hyperpigmentation) or be distributed in both areas (mixed hyperpigmentation). In the case of postinflammatory hypopigmentation, inflammatory mediators and cytokines are again involved in altering normal melanin synthesis and transfer. Severe inflammation can produce loss

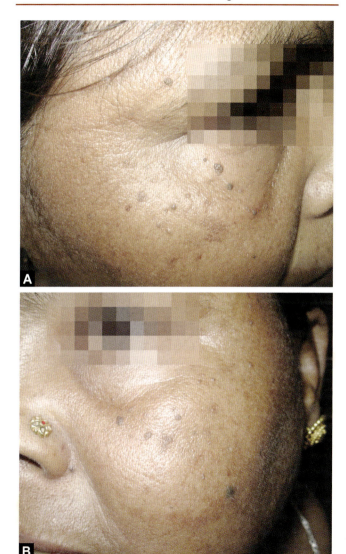

Figs 17.1A and B Photoaging in darker skins

of functional melanocytes, leading to hypo or depigmentation. The early treatment of inflammation in pigmented patients should be aggressive, to reduce pigmentary complications.

SUMMARY

- Pigmentary changes are more common and persistent
- Response to peeling agents can be unpredictable
- Demarcation lines are common
- Increased risk of hypertrophic scars and keloids
- Psychosocial and cosmetic distress is common due to marked changes in skin color
- Tropical climate leads to increased sun exposure.

Patient Assessment

Before attempting chemical peeling in skin of color, it is important to make a thorough evaluation of the patient. It is easier to fill a proforma so that no issues are missed. An extensive history should be taken at the first visit. Details of occupation and outdoor activities, including hobbies and games are essential to evaluate the quantum of sun exposure. One must assess whether the patient will be able to successfully avoid or reduce exposure to the sun following chemical peeling. Patients on photosensitizing drugs or suffering from photosensitive disorders are at higher risk of PIH, particularly in darker skin types. A past history of response of the skin to trauma, gives vital insights into the expected outcome of peels. Often patients give a history of persistent hyperpigmentation even on trivial trauma or repeated low grade trauma. This is commonly seen on the face in acne patients (Figure 17.2), on the arms due to insect bites or superficial burns in housewives and at friction sites such as the elbows in office workers, outer malleolus in people who squat on the floor and on the feet due to shoe bites. These areas should be examined carefully. A history of hypertrophic scars and keloids is a risk factor for medium and deep peels, but not usually for superficial peels.

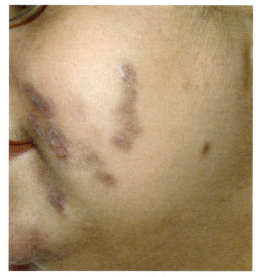

Fig. 17.2 Acne excoriée with hyperpigmentation

Careful selection of patients for chemical peeling should involve identification of Fitzpatrick skin type, and also determine ethnicity, as different ethnicities may respond unpredictably to chemical peeling regardless of skin phenotype. Ethnics with thick oily skin are better able to tolerate chemical peels as compared to patients with thin dry skin.

Counseling

Counseling the patient is very important prior to chemical peeling. The motivation and expectations of the patient should be judged. A media-hyped patient with unrealistic expectations invariably leads to dissatisfaction. Many darker skin patients expect dramatic lightening of skin color following chemical peels as a desired effect. This may occur transiently and may not be permanent. It is advisable to downplay the degree of improvement expected. Discussion about the nature of treatment, expected outcome, time taken for recovery of normal skin, likely complications, pigmentary changes and importance of maintenance regimens are essential. If the patient is not convinced, it is better to schedule another counseling session. The help of a professional counselor may be sought in case of problematic patients.

Priming and Preparation[3,4]

Priming with hypopigmenting agents should be done at least 4 to 6 weeks, before peeling. Hydroquinone 2 to 5% as tolerated, should be used. If hydroquinone causes irritation, alternative agents such as azelaic acid 10 to 20%, kojic acid 2%, arbutin 5% are alternative agents. Sun protection is very important and a combination of physical methods such as hats and umbrellas and chemical methods like broad spectrum sunscreens should be repeatedly advocated, particularly in patients with outdoor occupations. Glycolic acid 6 to 12% is useful as a priming agent in patients with thick uneven skin. Topical retinoids such as tretinoin 0.025 to 0.1%, adapalene 0.1% or tazarotene 0.5% should be used cautiously to avoid retinoid dermatitis and inflammation. The strength and duration of application of the priming agent should be increased gradually, if the patient has sensitive skin. Retinoids should be stopped 5 to 7 days before a peel, to prevent uneven or increased depth of peeling.

Precautions

Superficial chemical peels can be safely performed in dark skin patients.[5-15] However, medium and deep peels should be done with great caution, because of increased risk of pigmentary changes. Deep peels with phenol should be avoided due to the risk of permanent depigmentation, though there are few recent reports using modified phenol peels in darker skins.[16,17] Unlike deep peels, medium peels may be performed safely on people with olive and light brown skin, while the risk of discoloration is higher in patients with dark brown or black skin.[18,19] It is important to prepare the skin under medical supervision prior to peels. Superficial peels may give variable responses; hence a small test peel may be done in the postauricular or temple area to detect unpredictable responses to the peeling agent. This is particularly common with glycolic acid, trichloroacetic acid (TCA) and resorcinol. Lower concentration of the peeling agent should be first used and the concentration should be increased gradually, depending on response. All effort must be made to avoid excessive inflammation. It is safer to combine peels in lower concentrations to increase depth, rather than increase concentration of a single agent. One can also customize the peel to the individual face to get optimum results and avoid complications. Areas with thick, oily, damaged skin may require a deeper peel, while thinner, dry skin zones may only require a superficial peel.

Peel Selection

SAFE PEELS

- Glycolic acid 35 to 55%
- Mandelic acid 30 to 50%
- Salicylic acid 20 to 30%
- TCA 10 to 15%.

HIGH-RISK PEELS

- Jessner's peel (Lactic acid 14%, salicylic acid 14% with resorcinol 14 gm)
- TCA 25 to 35%
- Monheit's peel (Jessner's solution with 35% TCA)
- Coleman's peel (Glycolic acid 70% with TCA 35%).

PEELS BETTER AVOIDED

- Deep phenol peels.

Procedure

Familiarity with the properties of each peeling agent used is critical. The concentration of the peeling agent should be chosen with care. It is safer to choose a lower concentration and then titrate to a higher concentration after 1 to 2 peels. Spot peeling particularly with TCA gives good results and can avoid complications of peeling the entire face.[20] If greater depths of peeling are required, it is safer to combine lower concentrations of peeling agents rather than use high concentrations of single agents. For example, combining 35 to 70% glycolic acid for 3 minutes with TCA 15 to 25% is safer and effective as compared to 35% TCA used alone. Different procedures can also be combined. For example, combining CO_2 laser with TCA 25% or combining manual sand abrasion with 15% TCA.

Postpeel Care

The postpeel care is very important, to reduce risk of PIH. The patient should be adequately informed about the sequence of events after a chemical peel and how to take good care so as to reduce the chances of complications. Following a peel, any area of hyperpigmentation and scaling can show increased pigmentation initially, that can alarm the patient (Figure 17.3). This is more conspicuous in darker skins. It is part of normal peeling reaction and subsides when peeling is complete. Excessive inflammation should be treated with potent steroids like mometasone to prevent PIH.

Strict precautions for the patient during the healing phase should be observed.

- Avoid sun exposure as far as possible. Use physical measures like caps and umbrellas.

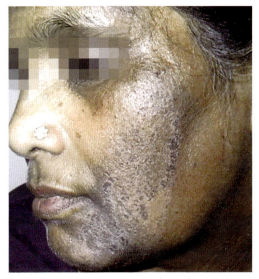

Fig. 17.3 Increased initial pigmentation after a peel with crusting

- Use broadspectrum sunscreens liberally and frequently.
- Do not pick, rub or peel the scales prematurely. Let them heal on their own.
- Start pretreatment priming agents as advised, particularly the hypopigmenting agents, to prevent PIH.
- The skin may be sensitive post peel and lower strengths of retinoids or glycolic acid should be used.
- Report immediately if there is delayed healing, persistent erythema, crusting or pain.

Complications

The best way to avoid complications is to identify patients at risk and use lighter peels. The deeper the peel, the greater is the risk of complications. Medium peels should be avoided or done with great precaution in type IV–VI skins. Patients at increased risk of complications are those with a history of postinflammatory hyperpigmentation, keloid formation, heavy occupational exposure to sun such as field workers, uncooperative patients and patients with a history of sensitive skin unable to tolerate sunscreens, hydroquinone, etc. Such patients should be closely followed up and if complications develop, they should be treated promptly and further peels should be stopped or postponed.

HYPERPIGMENTATION

Hyperpigmentation is very common, in patients with skin types IV–VI undergoing superficial or medium peels. It can occur any time after the peel and can be persistent, if inadequately treated. Though it can be triggered by sun exposure, it can also occur as an innate response in darker skin patients due to hyper-reactivity of the melanocytes, without significant sun exposure. Inflammation plays a key role in causing PIH due to release of cytokines that stimulate activity of melanocytes. Hence, controlling inflammation with topical and if required, systemic steroids becomes an essential part of postpeel care in dark skin patients. Bleaching agents like hydroquinone, kojic acid or azelaic acid combined with tretinoin or glycolic acid are useful for PIH. Repeeling with very superficial peels may give good response, if PIH persists beyond 2 to 4 weeks (Figures 17.4 and 17.5).

HYPOPIGMENTATION

A lighter and fairer complexion is normally seen after peeling and is much sought after by darker skin patients, where there is a craze for fairer complexions. This effect is transient in superficial peels due to sloughing off of the epidermis and removal of excess melanin. In medium peels, with removal of the basal layer, the hypopigmentation can be more prolonged,

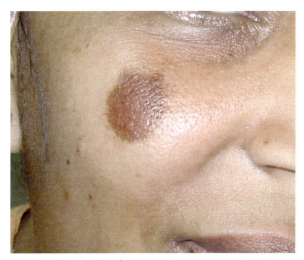

Fig. 17.4 Postinflammatory hyperpigmentation following glycolic acid peel 70%

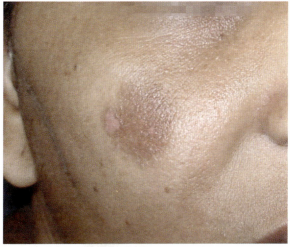

Fig. 17.5 PIH improving with topical steroid-mometasone

till melanocytes migrate from the surrounding skin and adnexae. In darker skins this hypopigmentation can be followed by PIH, due to overactivity of the melanocytes, hence medium peels are done with great caution in darker individuals. In deep peels, permanent hypopigmentation is common, which is not noticeable in fair type I and II skins, but can have disastrous consequences in darker skins. Hence deep peels are better avoided in darker skin types. Phenol, in addition, has a direct toxic effect on the melanocytes and can cause a permanent hypopigmentation with a peculiar alabaster look. If hypopigmentation is very noticeable, the untreated areas of the face and neck should be peeled to avoid lines of demarcation.

LINES OF DEMARCATION

These are lines of pigmentary change at the junction of peeled and unpeeled areas. They are common in all skin types and more common in darker skins and medium and deep peels. The periocular, perioral and jaw line are common sites of predilection. To avoid this, peeling agent with a lower concentration should be feathered at the edges to merge with the surrounding normal skin (Figure 17.6).

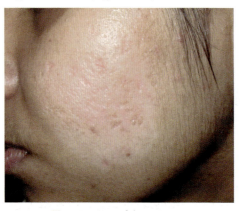

Fig. 17.6 Line of demarcation

Conclusion

Chemical peels are being commonly performed in darker racial-ethnic groups, individuals comprising skin types IV–VI, including Asians, Hispanics, Blacks, and Native Americans. Serial superficial glycolic acid, salicylic acid, Jessner's solution, and superficial TCA peels offer substantial benefits for post-inflammatory hyperpigmentation, melasma, acne, skin rejuvenation, pseudofolliculitis barbae, oily skin, and texturally rough skin. When selecting a peeling agent, the benefits of the procedure should always substantially outweigh any associated risks or complications, which are likely to be permanent. Superficial peels with lower concentrations are generally safe and efficacious for darker skinned patients. The concentrations should be gradually titrated to avoid severe inflammation and reaction. Topical steroids and hypopigmenting agents are invaluable in reducing PIH. Given the labile nature of melanocytes of darker complexioned individuals, medium-depth and deep peels are more likely to induce substantial complications and side effects, hence they are better avoided, particularly in skin types V and VI. It is important to note that hyperpigmentation occurring in light-skinned patients may last only a few weeks, whereas hyperpigmentation occurring in darker-skinned patients may last many months, years, or even a lifetime. In conclusion, chemical peeling, carefully performed can show excellent results in pigmentary and scarring disorders arising in dark skin tones.

Key Points

√ Superficial chemical peels can be safely performed in darker skin.
√ Prepeel priming is important to reduce the risk of complications.
√ Medium depth and deep peels can cause permanent pigmentary changes.
√ Complications peels in lower concentrations are safer and efficacious when repeated over a period of time.

References

1. Richards GM, Oresajo CO, Halder RM. Structure and function of ethnic skin and hair. Dermatol Clin. 2003;21:595-600.
2. Roberts WE. Chemical peeling in ethnic/dark skin. Dermatol Ther. 2004;17(2):196-205.
3. Nanda S, Grover C, Reddy BS. Efficacy of hydroquinone (2%) versus tretinoin (0.025%) as adjunct topical agents for chemical peeling in patients of melasma. Dermatol Surg. 2004;30(3):385-8; discussion 389.
4. Hexsel D, Arellano I, Rendon M. Ethnic considerations in the treatment of Hispanic and Latin-American patients with hyper-pigmentation. Br J Dermatol. 2006;156(Suppl 1):7-12.
5. Lim JT, Tham SN. Glycolic acid peels in the treatment of melasma among Asian women. Dermatol Surg. 1997;23(3):177-9.
6. Javaheri SM, Handa S, Kaur I, et al. Safety and efficacy of glycolic acid facial peel in Indian women with melasma. Int J Dermatol. 2001;40(5):354-7.
7. Sarkar R, Kaur C, Bhalla M, et al. The combination of glycolic acid peels with a topical regimen in the treatment of melasma in dark-skinned patients: A comparative study. Dermatol Surg. 2002;28(9):828-32; discussion 832.
8. Grover C, Reddu BS. The therapeutic value of glycolic acid peels in dermatology. Indian J Dermatol Venereol Leprol. 2003;69(2):148-50.
9. Cotellessa C, Peris K, Onorati MT, et al. The use of chemical peelings in the treatment of different cutaneous hyperpigmentations. Dermatol Surg. 1999;25(6):450-4.
10. Burns RL, Prevost-Blank PL, Lawry MA, et al. Glycolic acid peels for postinflammatory hyperpigmentation in black patients. A comparative study. Dermatol Surg. 1997;23(3):171-4: discussion 175.
11. Grimes PE. The safety and efficacy of salicylic acid chemical peels in darker racial-ethnic groups. Dermatol Surg. 1999;25(1):18-22.
12. Lee HS, Kim IH. Salicylic acid peels for the treatment of acne vulgaris in Asian patients. Dermatol Surg. 2003;29(12):1196-9; discussion 1199.
13. Bari AU, Iqbal Z, Rahman SB. Tolerance and safety of superficial chemical peeling with salicylic acid in various facial dermatoses. Indian J Dermatol Venereol Leprol. 2005;71(2):87-90.

14. Ahn HH, Kim IH. Whitening effect of salicylic acid peels in Asian patients. Dermatol Surg. 2006;32(3):372-5; discussion 375.
15. Khunger N, Sarkar R, Jain RK. Tretinoin peels versus glycolic acid peels in the treatment of Melasma in dark-skinned patients. Dermatol Surg. 2004;30(5):756-60; discussion 760.
16. Park JH, Choi YD, Kim SW, et al. Effectiveness of modified phenol peel (Exoderm) on facial wrinkles, acne scars and other skin problems of Asian patients. J Dermatol. 2007;34(1):17-24.
17. Yoon ES, Ahn DS. Report of phenol peel for Asians. Plast Reconstr Surg. 1999;103(1):207-14; discussion 215-7.
18. Kadhim KA, Al-Waiz M. Treatment of periorbital wrinkles by repeated medium-depth chemical peels in dark-skinned individuals. J Cosmet Dermatol. 2005;4(1):18-22.
19. Al-Waiz MM, Al-Sharqi AI. Medium-depth chemical peels in the treatment of acne scars in dark-skinned individuals. Dermatol Surg. 2002;28(5):383-7.
20. Chun EY, Lee JB, Lee KH. Focal trichloroacetic acid peel method for benign pigmented lesions in dark-skinned patients. Dermatol Surg. 2004;30:512-6; discussion 516.

18

Chemical Peeling in Sensitive Skin

Niti Khunger

- Problems
- Patient Assessment
- Counseling
- Priming and Preparation
- Precautions
- Peel Selection
- Procedure
- Postpeel Care
- Complications

Introduction

Sensitive skin is a term used to describe increased sensitivity of the skin, particularly on the face, to a wide range of external factors and products such as cosmetics including soaps and cleansers, heat, wind, climatic changes, spicy food and stress.[1,2] It is characterized by subjective symptoms like tingling, burning, irritation, tightness and cutaneous discomfort, without significant objective signs. There may be diffuse redness, dryness and irritation of the skin. However, sensitive skin may also be a marker for other skin disorders such as contact dermatitis, contact urticaria, atopic dermatitis, acne and rosacea. It is more commonly seen in patients who apply multiple cosmetic ingredients on the face, particularly scrubs, exfoliators, retinoids, alpha hydroxy acids (AHAs) and in those who undergo esthetic procedures like lasers, peels and skin abrasion.[3] In addition, when triggering agents continually bombard sensitive skin, they can cause premature skin aging, dryness, wrinkling, roughness, redness, and an unhealthy skin appearance. In such patients, choosing facial products and procedures is a real challenge. Many times these patients want treatment for persistent dyschromias and photoaging, where treatment can be frustrating.

Problems

- Sensitive skin cannot tolerate products such as sunscreens, retinoids, hydroquinone and glycolic acid used to prime the skin, before peeling.
- They usually have thin dry skin and chemical peels can penetrate deeper than intended, with greater risk of adverse effects.
- Sensitive skins react unpredictably to products used to maintain the effect of chemical peels.
- Repeated peelings can also make the skin more sensitive, particularly to heat while cooking and in hot sunny climates.

Patient Assessment

- Assess whether the patient will really benefit from the procedure.
- A detailed history of the cosmetic practices of the patient to uncover the causes of sensitive skin is essential.
- Evaluate the degree of sensitivity of the skin. If the patient has highly sensitive skin, chemical peeling should be deferred till the skin normalizes.
- Any subclinical underlying skin pathology such as contact dermatitis, contact urticaria, seborrheic dermatitis, atopic dermatitis and rosacea should be ruled out.
- Assess whether patient is likely to understand and follow postoperative instructions and report at the earliest, if any adverse event is suspected.

Counseling

Adequate counseling over repeated sessions is a must to justify whether the benefit of chemical peeling outweighs the risk associated with the procedure. The patient must be made to understand that results will not be dramatic, but occur gradually over a period of time. Serial peels can be stopped at any time due to unpredictable reactions of the skin. Likely complications and their treatment must be discussed.

Priming and Preparation

Priming of the skin is an important component of the procedure and must be undertaken cautiously in patients with sensitive skin as many products can be irritating. Sunscreens should contain only physical blockers such as zinc oxide or titanium dioxide, which are less likely to cause reactions. Chemical sunscreens should be avoided. Skin care regimen should be simple with a bland soap free cleanser like Cetaphil® and a mild moisturizer containing petrolatum or glycerin. Propylene glycol should be avoided as it can be an irritant. Priming products should contain single ingredients and be introduced one at a time with a gap of one week, so that the skin gets acclimatized and any unusual sensitivity can be detected. Retinoids should be used with extreme precaution. Adapalene is reported to be less irritating and should be preferred. Apply for a short duration, every alternate day and gradually increase the duration of application. If the skin is extremely dry use low strength tretinoin in cream base diluted with a moisturizer. In dark skins, a mild hypopigmenting agent such as arbutin, or low strength kojic acid is preferred. Most patients may not be able to tolerate hydroquinone. Glycolic acid should be avoided as it can increase sensitivity of the skin. Cosmetics should be perfume free and green tinted concealers may be used to mask redness.

Precautions

Before peeling, it must be emphasized that strict sun protection is essential. All factors that aggravate skin sensitivity should be avoided. Hot liquids or food, caffeine, spices, intense physical exercise and extreme temperatures (hot and cold) like saunas, and jacuzzis should be avoided. Underlying skin pathology and redness should first be treated, before attempting peeling. Mild topical corticosteroids like hydrocortisone 1% are beneficial, along with the use of bland moisturizers. Ideally a small test peel in the temple area should be done to check for unusual sensitivity and reaction of the skin to the peeling agent. During the peel, the lowest concentration should be initiated and peels should be spaced apart to give a chance for the skin to recover completely between peels. They should be deferred if the skin becomes unusually sensitive. Postpeel care should be meticulous, with strict sun protection, application of tolerated products and hypopigmenting agents. No new agents should be introduced. Complications should be detected at the earliest and promptly treated.

Peel Selection

Mild peels like lactic acid or mandelic acid are preferred over glycolic acid as they have a larger molecular weight and diffuse slowly into the skin. Lactic acid 40% is a mild superficial peel that can be used for sensitive skin.[4] It is useful for dyschromias and improving surface texture. Combined with arginine in gel form, it is useful for the treatment of photoaging in sensitive skin. (L-lactic acid 15%, arginine 20%, combined with 1% aloe vera and 0.5% allantoin Argipeel®).

Mandelic acid 30 to 40% is a superficial peel, useful in suppressing pigmentation, treating inflammatory noncystic acne, and rejuvenating photoaged skin. It is useful for acne due to its antibacterial properties.[5] The advantage of mandelic acid

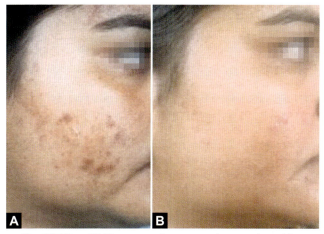

Figs 18.1A and B Treatment of postacne pigmentation with mandelic acid 40% in patient with sensitive skin

is that it does not cause stinging or burning on application and less erythema as compared to glycolic acid (Figures 18.1A and B).

In patients with extremely sensitive skins, lower concentrations of peeling agents combined together can be used, e.g. 15% mandelic acid/15% lactic acid or 30% mandelic acid/30% lactic acid or 30% mandelic acid/40% lactic acid.

Peels can also be used in gel formulations like the salicylic acid 20%, mandelic acid 10% with mediterranean fruit vinegar (Skin Ceuticals SM gel peel®). Salicylic acid in low concentration, 8% and 15% can also be used, particularly in patients with acne and in dark skins.

Glycolic acid in low concentrations 20 to 35% may be used cautiously in dark skin patients with sensitive skin. The exposure time should be increased very gradually.

Procedure

Detailed informed consent and photographic documentation are mandatory before peeling.

- The patient is asked to wash the face with a bland cleanser and water. The face is patted dry. It should not be rubbed.
- The hair is pulled back with a hairband or cap.
- The patient lies down with head elevated to 45° with eyes closed.
- Using 2″ × 2″ gauze pieces, the skin is cleaned gently with alcohol and then degreased gently with acetone or a prepeel cleanser which accompanies the kit.
- Sensitive areas of the face such as the lips, inner canthus of the eye and the nasolabial folds are protected with a thin layer of petrolatum.
- The concentration of the selected peeling agent is verified. It is poured in a glass cup and quickly applied using a cotton-tipped applicator or a brush or a gauze piece. Application is done in a predetermined manner to the facial cosmetic units, starting from the forehead and progressing to the cheeks, chin, perioral area, nose and lower eyelids. The whole procedure should be completed within 30 seconds.
- Feathering strokes are applied at the edges, to blend with surrounding skin and prevent demarcation lines.
- Do not leave the room. Watch out for unusual burning or hot spots. If they occur, that portion of the peel should be immediately terminated.
- At the endpoint, 1 to 3 minutes, the peel is terminated by washing with cold water.
- Patients are then sent home with a moisturizer and instructed to limit sun exposure and use sunscreens appropriately.

Postpeel Care

Patients feel tightness of the skin after a peel. Selected sunscreens and moisturizers are used postpeel till desquamation subsides. Mild soap or non-soap cleanser may be used. If there is crusting, topical antibacterial ointment should be used to prevent bacterial infection. They should avoid peeling or scratching the skin. A short course of systemic steroids, prednisolone 30 mg for 5 days, reduces inflammation and risk of side effects. If there is prolonged erythema, mid potency topical steroids like fluticasone or mometasone should be used for a short period. Hypopigmenting agents are restarted after the peeling subsides.

Intervals between the peels should be longer (4–6 weeks, in superficial peels) to give the skin sufficient time to recover between peels.

Complications

The best way to avoid complications in sensitive skin is to use lighter peels and good postpeel care. Severe burning may be experienced postpeel. This can be reduced by frequent applications of ice cold saline. Excessive crusting, desquamation, inflammation and erythema can occur. These should be treated aggressively to prevent postinflammatory hyperpigmentation (PIH), particularly in skins of color. Frequent applications of moisturizers, topical steroid cream like hydrocortisone 1% are used to reduce side effects. More potent steroids are used if there is severe irritation. The recovery of normal skin can take a longer time, up to 5 to 7 days.

Conclusion

The recent re-emergence of chemical peels and the availability of newer safer peeling agents have ensured that patients with sensitive skins can be safely peeled in experienced hands. It is better to err on the side of caution and use lower concentrations of peeling agents. Topical products should be chosen with care and underlying skin pathology should be treated before initiating chemical peeling in sensitive skin.

Key Points

√ Newer peels like mandelic acid and lactic acid have a larger molecular weight than glycolic acid, hence are slowly absorbed leading to fewer complications.
√ Topical skin products and peeling agents should be chosen with care.

References

1. Farage MA, Katsarou A, Maibach HI. Sensory, clinical and physiological factors in sensitive skin: a review. Contact Dermatitis. 2006;55(1):1-14.
2. R Jourdain, O. de Lacharrière, P Bastien, et al. Ethnic variations in self-perceived sensitive skin: epidemiological survey. Contact Dermatitis. 2002;46(3):162-9.
3. Baumann L. Cosmetic Dermatology: Principles and Practices. New York: McGraw-Hill, Medical Pub. Div. 2002.pp.33-9.
4. Sharquie KE, Al-Tikreety MM, Al-Mashhadani SA. Lactic acid chemical peels as a new therapeutic modality in melasma in comparison to Jessner's solution chemical peels. Dermatol Surg. 2006;32(12):1429-36.
5. Taylor MB. Summary of mandelic acid for the improvement of skin conditions. Cosmet Dermatol. 1999;12:28.

19

Chemical Peeling in Aging Skin

Niti Khunger

- Problems
- Patient Assessment
- Counseling
- Priming and Preparation
- Precautions
- Peel Selection
- Procedure
- Postpeel Care
- Complications

Introduction

A dramatic change in attitudes towards aging has led to an exponential increase in demand for antiaging therapies. In addition, due to depletion of ozone layer in the atmosphere, the exposure to harmful ultraviolet (UV) rays of the sun has increased, leading to skin aging becoming more common and evident in younger and younger individuals, in their twenties and thirties. The skin is a regenerative organ and can be stimulated to repair and renew itself. Hence, though aging is inevitable, skin rejuvenation techniques can partially reverse the effects of aging skin.

Skin aging is a complex biological process, governed by genetically programmed intrinsic factors causing atrophy of the epidermis, dermis, subcutaneous fat, muscle and bone, leading to fine wrinkles and lax skin with loss of elasticity.[1] Extrinsic aging is caused by prolonged sun exposure (photoaging), smoking, stress, and other environmental factors, leading to coarse dry skin, dyschromias, solar elastosis and deep wrinkles.

Chemical peels are one of the most frequently performed esthetic procedures and have re-emerged as popular, effective intervention techniques in the management of aging skin. The approach to peeling photoaging skin has now expanded beyond a single-stage procedure. Priming with medical therapy and post-treatment topical cosmeceutical therapy is essential to maintain results and prevent further photodamage. The physician should fully understand the nature of skin and degree of sun damage, techniques available, and active cosmeceutical agents that work for skin rejuvenation.

Problems

Mature skin is generally dry, thinner, sensitive and intolerant to many products. In addition, many geriatric patients are on systemic medications that can cause photosensitivity or pigmentation. These factors should be taken into account while selecting patients for chemical peels. Common problems seen in aging skin are (Figures 19.1 to 19.5):

- Fine and deep wrinkles
- Dyschromias
- Dry rough skin texture
- Surface growths
- Dilated pores
- Vascular lesions
- Skin laxity
- Loss of volume.

Patient Assessment

The assessment of the patient should be objective and clear, taking into account the age, ethnic variations and social

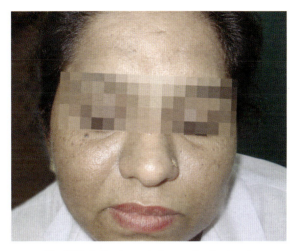

Fig. 19.1 Early pigmentation on the forehead, dermatosis papulosa skin (DPN), 30 years old

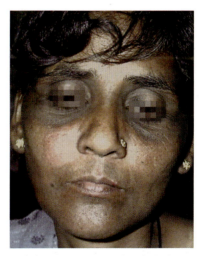

Fig. 19.2 Periorbital pigmentation with wrinkles, 40 years old

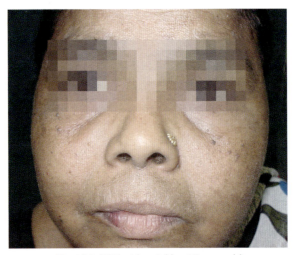

Fig. 19.3 DPN with wrinkles, 50 years old

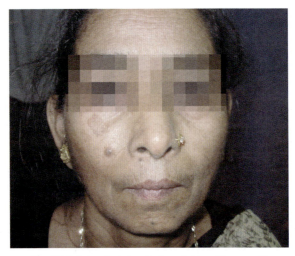

Fig. 19.4 Seborrheic keratosis, wrinkles, 60 years old

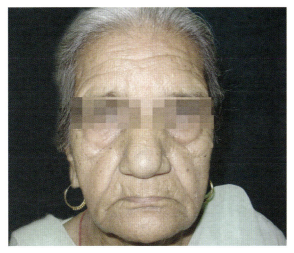

Fig. 19.5 Deep wrinkles, 70 years old

acceptability. Often conditions what the physician feels require therapeutic intervention, may be acceptable to the patient and vice versa.

A clinical assessment is done of each cosmetic unit and treatment planned accordingly. While analyzing the patient with photoaging skin, skin color and skin type as well as degree of photoaging is essential to select the right peel. Note the type of wrinkles, fine (hardly visible at rest, more visible with muscle movement), and deep (visible at rest, direction parallel or perpendicular to muscle activity). In darker skins, dyschromias in the form of lentigines or age spots, perioral and periorbital pigmentation, melasma, phototoxic melanosis, dermatosis papulosa nigra and seborrheic keratoses become more common. Macular amyloidosis, pseudoacanthosis nigricans, pigmentary demarcation lines, and facial melanosis like Riehls melanosis are more common signs of skin aging. The skin becomes dry, rough and sallow, with dilated pores.

Achrocordons or skin tags are commonly seen on the neck and axilla, particularly in obese persons. Vascular lesions in the form of telangiectasia, cherry spots, and rosacea like lesions become apparent.

A psychological assessment is also important. The problem areas from the patient's point of view should be targeted and a realistic appraisal of the expected outcomes should be given to the patient. Patients with body dysmorphobic disorders, depression, and psychotic conditions should be avoided.

Counseling

Adequate counseling is the cornerstone for a successful skin rejuvenation program. The patient must be clearly informed about the limitations of the procedure and expected outcomes must be lowered to avoid unsatisfied patients. The alternatives to treatment must be discussed and time taken for recovery of normal skin. Complications in particular pigmentary changes in darker skins must be spelt out and the importance of proper prepeel and postpeel care. Superficial peels are not one time procedures, but require multiple sessions and maintenance therapy. Superficial chemical peeling is effective only for surface skin damage. The effects of aging in deeper tissues, such as sagging jowls and drooping eyelids, must be addressed by other procedures.

Priming and Preparation

A priming regimen should be followed before peeling, to enhance results and reduce risk of complications. Mature patients usually have dry thin skins; hence sunscreens with moisturizers are useful in the daytime. Topical retinoids, tretinoin 0.05% or isotretinoin 0.5% in cream base are proved therapeutic agents for the treatment of aging skin. Topical retinoids improve skin texture, dyschromias and fine lines on prolonged usage and are an essential part of any skin rejuvenation program. Retinoid dermatitis is common in patients with mature dry and sensitive skin; hence it should be initially applied for short duration or alternate days, till tolerance develops. Less irritating formulations like microsphere encapsulated or low strength cream formulations are better tolerated. Low strength alpha hydroxy acids (AHAs) like glycolic acid are proven remedies for aging skin. They improve surface texture and also cause increase of collagen and ground substance in the dermis. Topical hypopigmenting agents are necessary in darker skins, to reduce the risk of post-inflammatory hyperpigmentation (PIH).

Precautions

Pigmentary changes are risk factors in skin of color. The problem is less with very superficial and superficial chemical peels, but may become a significant problem with medium and deep chemical peels in darker skins. These peels can also be a significant risk with regional areas with thin skin such as lips, perioral region and eyelids, are peeled deeply, with potential for scarring and significant changes in color. It can lead to conspicuous color mismatch in these cosmetic units from the rest of the face. The physician must be careful in doing deeper peels, especially in skin types III–VI. Deeper chemical peels must be performed only if the benefits of the procedure outweigh these risks. Many older patients are on systemic medications, such as antidiabetics, antihypertensives, antidepressants, antipsychotics, painkillers including nonsteroidal anti-inflammatory drugs (NSAIDs) that are photosensitizing or can cause increased pigmentation. These patients are at increased risk for pigmentary complications occurring following chemical peels. Peels must be avoided or done with extreme caution in these patients. Strict sun protection and appropriate techniques to prevent these unwanted changes in color must be emphasized.

Peel Selection[2-10]

Superficial chemical peels, often called lunchtime peels are useful for dyschromias, superficial growths like seborrheic and actinic keratosis, dermatoses papulosa nigra and for improving skin texture. Young patients with minimal skin damage often respond best to a series of light superficial peels in combination with a skin care program. Glycolic acid 35 to 70% applied for 3 to 5 minutes is the most widely used superficial peeling agent for aging skin (*see* Figure 19.2). Trichloroacetic acid (TCA) 10 to 15% is particularly useful in patients with rough texture and superficial growths (*see* Figure 19.3). Salicylic acid 20 to 30% is appropriate for patients with thick oily acne prone skin (*see* Figure 19.4). Tretinoin peels 1 to 5% have also been used for photoaging (*see* Figure 19.5). Lactic acid peels 40 to 50% are useful for dry sensitive skins and in patients with rosacea. Kojic acid inhibits the catecholase activity of tyrosinase and is used as a lightening agent. A gel solution composed of 50% glycolic acid and 10% kojic acid was reported to be useful in the treatment of hyperpigmentation and photoaging. It may be particularly useful for patients with prominent pigmentary changes.

Medium depth peels are effective for older patients with moderate skin damage, including surface growths, dilated pores and fine lines. A medium-depth peel may be combined with another treatment such as laser resurfacing to achieve maximum benefit. Glycolic acid 50 to 70% applied for 3 to 10 minutes, TCA 25% are safer for skin of color. In selected patients, a 20 to 35% TCA peel can dramatically diminish fine lines and wrinkles, remove sun damage, even skin tone and change the rougher texture of the upper eyelids, resulting in younger looking eyes.

It is safer to combine peels, using lower strengths than higher concentrations. For example, glycolic acid 70% plus TCA 35% or Jessner's solution plus TCA 35%. Pyruvic acid, an alpha ketoacid, induces both epidermal and dermal effects by diminishing the cohesion of epidermal corneocytes leading to thinning of the epidermis, and increasing production of collagen, elastic fibers and glycoproteins causing thickening of the dermis. The patients treated with pyruvic acid 50% reported very limited or no discomfort in the postpeel period. Hence, pyruvic acid was proposed as a safe and efficient treatment for moderate facial skin aging. Mandelic acid 30 to 40% is also useful as a safe peeling agent in darker skins. Studies have shown improvement in photoaged skin, acne, abnormal pigmentation, and skin texture with mandelic acid 40% peels.

Deep peels help to an extent in treating deeper wrinkles in patients with skin type I–III. They should be performed only by experienced physicians as there is a very low margin of safety in such peels. They are avoided in skin types IV–VI due to a significant risk of permanent hypopigmentation developing in these patients. Chemical peeling will obviously not help in the treatment of vascular lesions, skin laxity and loss of volume. The selection of the peeling agent and strength is individualized according to the skin type and degree of damage. It can be different in different cosmetic units and change over a period of time, according to requirement.

Procedure

Detailed informed consent and photographic documentation are mandatory before peeling.

- The patient is asked to wash the face with a bland cleanser and water. The face is patted dry. It should not be rubbed.
- The hair are pulled back with a hairband or cap.
- The patient lies down with head elevated to 45° with eyes closed.
- Using 2″ × 2″ gauze pieces, the skin is cleaned gently with alcohol and then degreased with acetone or a prepeel cleanser which accompanies the kit.
- Sensitive areas of the face such as the lips, inner canthus of the eye and the nasolabial folds are protected with a thin layer of petrolatum.

- Any superficial growth such as seborrheic keratosis dermatosis papulosa nigra are first removed with radio-frequency or CO_2 laser.
- The concentration of the selected peeling agent is verified. It is poured in a glass cup and quickly applied using a cotton-tipped applicator or a brush or a gauze piece. Application is done in a predetermined manner to the facial cosmetic units, starting from the forehead and progressing to the cheeks, chin, perioral area, nose and lower eyelids. The whole procedure should be completed within 30 seconds.
- Feathering strokes are applied at the edges, to blend with surrounding skin and prevent demarcation lines.
- Watch out for unusual burning or hot spots. If they occur that portion of the peel should be immediately terminated.
- At the endpoint, the peel is terminated by washing with cold water.
- Patients are then sent home with a moisturizer and instructed to limit sun exposure and use sunscreens appropriately.

Postpeel Care

Patients feel tightness of the skin after a peel. Selected sunscreens and moisturizers are used postpeel till desquamation subsides. Healing may be delayed in older skins. Mild soap or non-soap cleanser may be used. If there is crusting, topical antibacterial ointment should be used to prevent bacterial infection as older patients are much more prone to infection. They should avoid peeling or scratching the skin. A short course of systemic steroids, prednisolone 30 mg for 5 days, reduces inflammation and risk of side effects. If here is prolonged erythema mid potency topical steroids like fluticasone or mometasone should be used. Hypopigmenting agents are restarted after the peel.

Superficial peels can be repeated every 2 weeks, medium depth peels may be repeated after 6 to 9 months, while deep peels should not be repeated before one year.

Complications

The best way to avoid complications in aging skin is to use combination peels or combinant procedures for maximum effect with minimal risks. Skin that has been conditioned prior to a chemical peel will heal faster with fewer complications. Strict sun protection and good postpeel care are important. Severe burning may be experienced postpeel. This can be reduced by frequent applications of ice cold saline. Skin irritation, infection, scarring, flare up of herpes, worsening of the treated problem (mostly seen with melasma) as well as pigmentary abnormalities are the most common problems that are seen following medium depth chemical peels. Excessive crusting, desquamation, inflammation and erythema can occur with all peels. These should be treated aggressively to prevent PIH, particularly in skins of color. Frequent application of moisturizers, topical steroid cream like hydrocortisone 1% are used to reduce side effects. More potent steroids are used if there is severe irritation. The skin returns to normal in superficial peels in 2 to 5 days and in 7 to 10 days in medium peels.

Conclusion

Chemical peels are popular methods of skin rejuvenation because they are versatile, offer significant benefit with minimum downtime. The choice of peeling agents can be varied according to skin type, offering a good safety profile in experienced hands. Besides they are maintenance free as no instrumentation is required and they can be performed as out-patient procedures. It is the obligation of the physician to analyze the patient's skin type and the degree of photoaging skin, and thus prescribe the correct facial rejuvenation procedure. Any interventional procedure or combination of procedures that will give the greatest benefit for the least risk factors and morbidity should be selected. Though chemical peeling has been the true basic procedure for treatment of aging skin, the peeling agent and its strength should be chosen carefully to minimize risks. It is the responsibility of the physician to choose the correct modality to treat photoaging skin, scars, dyschromias, and the removal of skin growths, taking into account ethnic and social factors, skin type and overall general health of the patient rather than being influenced by the media-hyped patient. The physician must have thorough knowledge of all of these tools to give each patient the correct treatment. It has been rightly said that the art and science of chemical peeling is re-emerging, as one of the most effective ways to combat skin aging.

Key Points

√ Photoaging in darker skins predominantly manifests as dyschromias in the form of lentigines or age spots, perioral and periorbital pigmentation, melasma, phototoxic melanosis, dermatosis papulosa nigra and seborrheic keratoses. Macular amyloidosis, pseudo-acanthosis nigricans, pigmentary demarcation lines, and facial melanoses like Riehls melanosis are other common signs of skin aging, apart from wrinkles. The skin becomes dry, rough and sallow, with dilated pores.

√ Superficial chemical peels are useful for dyschromias, superficial growths like seborrheic and actinic keratosis, dermatoses papulosa nigra and for improving skin texture.

√ Young patients with minimal skin damage often respond best to a series of light superficial peels in combination with a skin care program.

√ Medium depth peels are effective for older patients with moderate skin damage, including surface growths, dilated pores and fine lines. A medium-depth peel may be combined with another treatment such as laser resurfacing to achieve maximum benefit.

√ Deep peels help to an extent in treating deeper wrinkles in patients with skin type I–III. They should be performed only by experienced physicians as there is a very low margin of safety in such peels. They are avoided in skin types IV–VI due to a significant risk of permanent hypopigmentation developing in these patients.

√ Chemical peeling will obviously not help in the treatment of vascular lesions, skin laxity and loss of volume. The selection of the peeling agent and strength is individualized according to the skin type and degree of damage. It can be different in different cosmetic units and change over a period of time, according to requirement.

References

1. Rabe JH, Mamelak AJ, McElgunn PJ, et al. Photoaging: Mechanisms and repair. J Am Acad Dermatol. 2006;55(1):1-19. Review.
2. Roenigk HH Jr. Treatment of the aging face. Dermatol Clin. 1995;13(2):245-61. Review.
3. Chun EY, Lee JB, Lee KH. Focal trichloroacetic acid peel method for benign pigmented lesions in dark-skinned patients. Dermatol Surg. 2004;30:512-6.
4. Vedamurthy M. Salicylic acid peels. Indian J Dermatol Venereol Leprol. 2004;70:136-8.
5. Ghersetich I, Brazzini B, Peris K, et al. Pyruvic acid peels for the treatment of photoaging. Dermatol Surg. 2004;30(1):32-6.
6. Taylor MB. Summary of mandelic acid for the improvement of skin conditions. Cosmet Dermatol. 1999;12:28.
7. Fulton JE, Rahimi D, Helton P, et al. Neck rejuvenation by combining Jessner/TCA peel, dermasanding, and CO_2 laser resurfacing. Dermatol Surg. 1999;25:745-50.
8. Fulton JE, Porumb S. Chemical peels: Their place within the range of resurfacing techniques. Am J Clin Dermatol. 2004;5(3):179-87. Review.
9. Moy LS, Murad H, Moy RL. Glycolic acid peels for the treatment of wrinkles and photoaging. J Dermatol Surg Oncol. 1993;19(3):243-6.
10. Manaloto RM, Alster TS. Periorbital rejuvenation: A review of dermatologic treatments. Dermatol Surg. 1999;25(1):1-9. Review.

20

Chemical Peels in Acne and Acne Scars

Niti Khunger

- Problems in Acne that can be Treated with Chemical Peels
- Counseling
- Priming and Preparation
- Precautions
- Peel Selection
- Procedure
- Technique
- Postpeel Care
- Complications

Introduction

Chemical peels are being increasingly used for active acne. The basic aim is prevention and reduction in the severity of scarring. If done correctly, then they can prevent or reduce the incidence and severity of permanent postacne scars by early reduction in comedones, quicker resolution of inflammation and treatment of postinflammatory pigmentation. They can also reduce oiliness of the skin and help in improvement of superficial scars.

Traditionally, medium depth and deep peels were carried out for the treatment of acne scars. Trichloroacetic acid (TCA) and phenol were the common agents used. However, medium depth and deep peels carry a higher risk of complications, particularly in darker skins, and they have been largely supplanted by fractional lasers. Still, repeated superficial chemical peels can play an active role in the treatment of persistent macular hyperpigmented and erythematous lesions and superficial acne scars. An advantage of chemical peels is that can be utilized in the presence of active acne lesions and also help to improve pigmentary dyschromias, photoaging and texture of the skin.

Problems in Acne that Can be Treated with Chemical Peels

- Excessive oiliness
- Comedones—open and closed
- Persistent postinflammatory hyperpigmentation in darker skins
- Persistent erythematous scars
- Superficial atrophic scars.

Superficial chemical peels ablate the epidermis; this exfoliation reduces comedones and also helps in the treatment of pigmented macular scars. Exfoliation is followed by epidermal regeneration and collagen formation in the dermis. Because they are mildly potent, repeated treatments are required to obtain the desired effects. They are predominantly useful in macular and mild atrophic scars (superficial boxcar scars).

Medium depth chemical peels extend to the papillary dermis. The inflammatory reaction has stimulatory effects on fibroblasts resulting in new collagen formation. This explains their efficacy on atrophic scars.

For atrophic scars better results are obtained if they are combined with subcision. The subcision is done first, followed by the chemical peel. It can be used when patient has active acne. It also leads to improvement of skin texture and pigmentation.

Counseling

This is very important prior to chemical peeling. Proper and adequate counseling is the most effective method to prevent patient dissatisfaction and calm down a patient, if complications occur. The physician should assess the motivation and expectations of the patient and downplay the degree of improvement expected. The time taken for recovery of normal skin, likely complications, pigmentary changes that can occur should be clearly explained. The importance of maintenance regimens after the peel should be emphasized.

Priming and Preparation

Priming is preparation of the skin before peeling. It decreases risk of post-inflammatory hyperpigmentation, reduces wound healing time, facilitates uniform penetration of peeling agent, detects intolerance of any agent and most important, enforces patient compliance for following instructions in the postpeel period.

The patient should be primed with skin lightening agents such as hydroquinone 2%, tretinoin 0.025% or adapalene 0.1% at least 2 to 4 weeks before the procedure. Triple combination creams containing steroids should be strictly avoided as it can lead to aggravation of acne. Sun exposure should be avoided and sunscreens regularly applied. Antivirals should be given two days prior in patients with history of herpes simplex. Topical retinoids should be stopped 2 to 3 days before planning a peel to avoid irritation.

Precautions

One must have a conservative approach in treating acne with chemical peels. Aggressive peeling can lead to increased inflammation and adverse effects. Peels should be performed cautiously in patients with a history of herpes simplex. During active lesions, the peels should be deferred. It is safer to treat the herpes simplex with antivirals and then do the peels under the cover of prophylactic antivirals starting two days prior to the procedure and continuing for a week after the peel. Viral infections such as warts or molluscum contagiosum on the area to be peeled should first be treated. Open wounds or excoriations that can occur in acne excoriee should not be peeled as it can lead to increased penetration of the peel followed by scarring. Chemical peels should be performed with caution in patients on photosensitive drugs, particularly doxycycline and minocycline as they can lead to greater and persistent erythema, followed by postinflammatory hyperpigmentation.

Patients on isotretinoin or with a history of use in the last six months can safely undergo superficial peels. However, deep peels should be avoided.

Patients who do not apply the sunscreen and medications as frequently as prescribed or are careless about sun exposure should be cautiously taken up for chemical peels. They have higher chances of pigmentary complications, which can worsen the clinical condition.

Patient with unrealistic expectations are also poor candidates. Superficial chemical peels are useful only for macular and mild superficial atrophic acne scars. They are not useful for deeper icepick and boxcar scars or in patient with extensive atrophy, which should be clearly explained to the patient.

Peel Selection

A wide variety of peeling agents can be used for active acne.
- Salicylic acid 20 to 30% lotion or gel
- Mandelic acid 40 to 50% lotion or gel
- Retinoid peels (Yellow peel)
- Lactic acid 60 to 90%
- Glycolic acid 20 to 70%

- Modified Jessner's solution—14% salicylic acid, 14% lactic acid, 14% citric acid
- TCA 15 to 35%
- Pyruvic acid 40 to 60%.

Salicylic acid 20% to 30% is the peeling agent of choice in active acne since it has keratolytic and anti-inflammatory properties. Being lipophilic in nature, it can easily penetrate the pilosebaceous apparatus (Figures 20.1A to C).

Mandelic acid is good for pustular lesions since it has antibacterial properties. Acne with pigmentation, acne with melasma and acne excoriee are ideal situations to use mandelic acid peels. For chemical peeling 30%, 40% or 50%

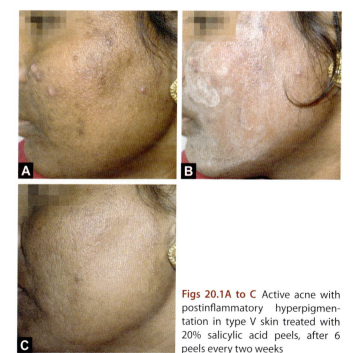

Figs 20.1A to C Active acne with postinflammatory hyperpigmentation in type V skin treated with 20% salicylic acid peels, after 6 peels every two weeks

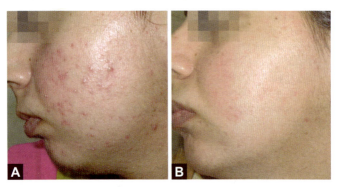

Figs 20.2A and B Active acne with sensitive skin, intolerant to topical retinoids and benzoyl peroxide treated with combination salicylic-mandelic acid peels in a gel base

mandelic acid is safer in darker skin types as well as in those with sensitive skin.

Combination peels, particularly salicylic-mandelic acid combination in lotion or gel forms are excellent peels for active acne[1] (Figures 20.2A and B). The lotion form is used for oily skins and the gel based are used for sensitive, dry or erythematous skins. If patient is prone to PIH, the initial peeling agent should be of lower strength and the gradually strength should be increased or combination peels should be used.

Retinoid peels are excellent for patients with thick oily skin and acne grade 1 with lot of comedones (Figures 20.3A and B). They should be used cautiously in patients with sensitive dry skin as they can cause a lot of exfoliation, which can lead to PIH.

Lactic acid is a good peeling agent during pregnancy when most anti-acne medications are contraindicated. A study utilizing full strength 92% lactic acid in 7 patients with Fitzpatrick skin type IV-V showed it to be safe with modest improvement.[2]

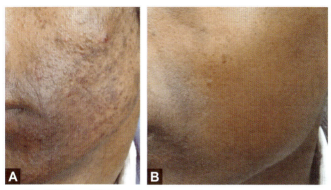

Figs 20.3A and B Comedonal acne with pigmentation treated with yellow peel in type V skin

The peeling agent should be carefully selected in patients with active acne to avoid complications (Table 20.1).

Combination peels containing salicylic acid, mandelic acid, retinol, citric acid, kojic acid are advocated. For superficial atrophic scars peels containing glycolic acid 35 to 70 %,[3] pyruvic acid 40 to 60%[4] or TCA 15 to 25% should be used. They can be combined with subcision and microneedling. Chemical peels should not be utilized for deep scarring, that extends beyond the papillary dermis, such as icepick scars and deep boxcar scars. The high strength TCA CROSS technique is a focal deep modified form of a chemical peel used for icepick scars.[5]

A modified phenol peel Exoderm® has also been used in Asian patients with acne scars.[6] Though an improvement was observed in 7 out of 11 patients (64%), postinflammatory hyperpigmentation was observed in 74% and 1 patient developed persistent hypopigmentation. Hence, phenol peels are better avoided in darker skin types, besides the risk of cardiac arrythmias. The newer combination peels have multiple modes of action and have a wide margin of safety. They may require more sessions and may be only moderately effective.

Table 20.1: Selection of peels in acne

Type of acne/acne scars	Choice of peel
Active acne grade 1—comedones	Salicylic acid 20–30% Retinol peel 5% Glycolic acid 20–35 %
Active acne grade 2—papules/pustules	Salicylic acid 20–30% Mandelic acid 40–50%
Active acne grade 3—pustules	Salicylic acid 20–30% Mandelic acid 40–50%
Pigmented acne scars	Combination peels with salicylic acid, mandelic acid, kojic acid, citric acid Retinol peel (Yellow peel) Jessner's peel
Persistent erythematous scars	Salicylic acid 20% Mandelic acid 20%
Superficial atrophic scars	Glycolic acid 35–70% TCA 15–25% Pyruvic acid 50%
Icepick scars	TCA CROSS 50–100%
Acne in pregnancy	Lactic acid 70–90%

Technique

Informed consent and documentation with photographs are important prerequisites. Contact lenses should be removed before the peel. The patient washes the face with soap and water to remove all makeup, dirt and grime and the hair is pulled back with a hairband or cap.

The patient is either sitting or inclined at 45 degrees. The skin is cleaned with a prepeel cleanser and oily skins are degreased with acetone. The peeling agent of required strength is poured in a glass beaker and the neutralizing agent is kept ready. The agent is applied with a cotton tipped applicator on the entire face going along the cosmetic units. There should be no dripping of the agent. Begin from the forehead in an upward direction, then the right cheek, nose, left cheek and chin in that order. Feathering strokes are applied at the edges, to blend with surrounding skin and prevent demarcation lines. In grade 1 acne with plenty of comedones, comedone extraction is done first followed by the chemical peel. If the comedones are difficult to extract, undue pressure should not be used. Two to three glycolic acid peels 20 to 35% done every fortnight will cause comedolysis and make comedone extraction easier.

Do not leave the room and closely watch out for increasing redness, hot spots and epidermolysis. The peel is neutralized as required according to the peeling agent. The skin is gently dried with gauze and the patient is asked to wash with cold water till the burning subsides. The patient then applies a sunscreen, before leaving the clinic. A gel base peel or a retinol peel are leave on peels for 6 to 8 hours, hence are not neutralized.

Postpeel Care

Patients may feel tightness of the skin after a peel or may show frank desquamation, especially after the first peel. Following a retinol peel (yellow peel) exfoliation or peeling of the skin occurs after 2 to 3 days and can last for 2 to 5 days. They should be prepared for this. A sunscreen in aqueous base should be used. If required, a non-comedogenic moisturizer may be used postpeel if the patient is uncomfortable. Healing may be delayed in older skins and in patients with many atrophic scars. A mild soap or non-soap cleanser may be used. If there is crusting, topical antibacterial ointment should be used to prevent bacterial infection as older patients are much more prone to infection. Patients should be emphatically told to avoid peeling or scratching the skin. Topical anti-acne medications are withheld after the peel till exfoliation is completed. They are restarted when the patient feels a smooth natural feel to the skin. Superficial peels can be repeated every 2 weeks. Medium depth peels may be repeated after 6 to 9 months, while deep peels should not be repeated before one year.

COMBINATION TREATMENTS

The advantage of chemical peels is that they can be combined with other modalities like subcision, microneedling and fractional lasers for an additive effect. While subcision and microneedling take care of the atrophy in the dermis, chemical peels improve the surface texture of the skin. When combining chemical peels with subcision, the subcision is done first, followed by the peel. If combing with microneedling, the chemical peel is done first or the two modalities can be used alternatively, every two weeks.

Complications

The best way to avoid complications during peeling, particularly in patients with acne is to use combination peels. A well primed skin will heal faster with fewer complications. Strict sun protection and good postpeel care are important. Severe burning may be experienced postpeel, especially over active lesions. This can be reduced by frequent applications of ice cold saline. Complications with superficial peels are uncommon (Table 20.2). Postinflammatory hyperpigmentation is most frequently seen, particularly if the patient has not been primed with skin lightening agents or there is excessive prolonged peeling combined with retinoid dermatitis. Skin irritation, infection, aggravation of acne, flare up of herpes, and pigmentary abnormalities are complications that can occur following medium depth chemical peels. Excessive crusting, desquamation, inflammation and erythema can occur with all peels. These should be treated aggressively to prevent PIH, particularly in skins of color. Short course of mild topical steroid, like hydrocortisone can be prescribed for 2 to 4 days to tide over the inflammatory phase, only if it is very severe. The skin returns to normal in superficial peels in 2 to 5 days and in 7 to 10 days in medium peels.

| Table 20.2: Complication of peels and their management ||
Problem	Solution
Aggravation of acne	Put patient on oral antibiotics
Too many comedones	Comedone extraction, followed by peels
Comedones difficult to extract	Apply mild glycolic or TCA peel, followed 2 weeks later by comedone extraction
Peel shows no effect	Rule out underlying causes
Patient on isotretinoin	Can do superficial peels Avoid medium depth peels Avoid high strength glycolic acid and TCA peels
Recurrence of acne	Continue maintenance treatment
Patient develops PIH	Stop peel, give sunscreens, topical hydroquinone, kojic acid, arbutin
Patient develops persistent erythema	Sign of overpeeling, stop retinoids. Advise regular sunscreen use

Key Points

√ Chemical peels are useful adjunctive procedures for active acne, for erythematous and hyperpigmented macular acne scars, acne excoriee and atrophic mild superficial scars.

√ Additive improvement occurs when they are combined with other procedures such as subcision, microneedling, fractional lasers and CROSS technique.

√ They are a useful adjunct when patient has active acne, photo-damage and postinflammatory hyperpigmentation.

√ Salicylic acid, mandelic acid, glycolic acid, Jessner's solution and TCA are peeling agents of choice used, singly or as combination peels.

References

1. Garg VK, Sinha S, Sarkar R. Glycolic acid peels versus salicylic-mandelic acid peels in active acne vulgaris and post-acne scarring and hyperpigmentation: a comparative study. Dermatol Surg. 2009;35:59-65.

2. Sachdeva S. Lactic acid peeling in superficial acne scarring in Indian skin. J Cosmet Dermatol. 2010;9(3):246-8.

3. Erbağci Z, Akçali C. Biweekly serial glycolic acid peels vs. long-term daily use of topical low-strength glycolic acid in the treatment of atrophic acne scars. Int J Dermatol. 2000;39(10):789-94.

4. Al-Waiz MM, Al-Sharqi AI. Medium-depth chemical peels in the treatment of acne scars in dark-skinned individuals. Dermatol Surg. 2002;28(5):383-7

5. Park JH, Choi YD, Kim SW, et al. Effectiveness of modified phenol peel (Exoderm) on facial wrinkles, acne scars and other skin problems of Asian patients. J Dermatol. 2007;34(1):17-24.

6. Khunger N. IADVL Task Force. Standard guidelines of care for chemical peels. Indian J Dermatol Venereol Leprol. 2008;74 Suppl:S5-12.

21

Chemical Peels in Melasma and Facial Melanoses

Niti Khunger

- Problems in Facial Melanoses
- Patient Assessment and Counseling
- Priming and Preparation
- Precautions
- Peel Selection
- Procedure
- Postpeel Care
- Complications

Introduction

Melasma is a very common cause of facial pigmentation, particularly in darker skins. Other common causes include post inflammatory hyperpigmentation (PIH), pigmented cosmetic dermatitis (Riehl's melanosis), actinic lichen planus, lichen planus pigmentosis, pigmentary demarcation lines and photosensitive dermatoses. Facial melanoses are difficult to treat as many of them are dermal with melanophages in the dermis (Table 21.1). The problems associated with management are that often the etiology is difficult to detect, there is a lack of effective treatment modalities, aggressive treatment can worsen the pigmentation and recurrences are common. Triple combination creams though effective, cannot be prescribed for long periods due to their adverse effects. Chemical peels offer an alternate treatment modality in hyperpigmented skin disorders.

Table 21.1: Pathogenetic classification of facial pigmentation		
Epidermal	*Dermal*	*Mixed (Epidermal and Dermal)*
Melasma	Nevus of Ota	Melasma
Ephelides	Hori's nevus	Pigmented cosmetic
Solar lentigines		dermatitis
PIH		Periorbital melanosis
		Solar lentigines
		Poikiloderma
		Fixed drug eruptions
		Actinic lichen planus
		Ashy dermatosis
		PIH
		Exogenous ochronosis

Abbreviation: PIH: Postinflammatory hyperpigmentation

They act by causing exfoliation, hence reducing epidermal pigmentation and reducing epidermal turnover time.

Problems in Facial Melanoses

Chemical peels should be cautiously performed in facial pigmentation as aggressive treatment can worsen pigmentation due to PIH. There is a very small margin of safety, particularly in darker skins. Patient should be adequately primed before starting peels. Recurrences are common, hence maintenance treatment is essential.

Patient Assessment and Counseling

The diagnosis of melasma is usually straightforward. However diagnosis of other causes of facial pigmentation may not be obvious and can be arrived at after careful history and examination. A detailed history regarding usage of products on the face should be undertaken. Treating the pigmentation with chemical peels becomes a futile exercise if the causative agent is not eliminated. The degree and duration of sun exposure, precipitating factors like hormones, contraceptive pills, perfumed or colored cosmetics and photosensitizing medications or products used including Ayurvedic, Homeopathic and home remedies should be assessed. On examination if the pigmentation is brownish it is more likely to be epidermal, whereas a bluish-gray pigmentation is more likely to be dermal. On Wood's lamp examination, epidermal pigmentation will get enhanced and dermal pigmentation will show no change. But this is useful mainly in fair skins Type I–IV.

Dermoscopy and finally a skin biopsy is the best technique to determine depth of pigmentation. The patient must be clearly informed about the limitations of treatment that can occur with chemical peels and the incidence of recurrences. Probable complications and how to deal with them must be discussed honestly. The importance of adequate sun protection must be emphasized at every visit.

Priming and Preparation

A priming regimen given in writing to the patient is essential before peeling. Effective sunscreens are the most important tools to prevent recurrences. They must be consistently and regularly applied. Retinoids, low strength glycolic acid 10% along with hydroquinone 2 to 5% or kojic acid 2% are used as priming agents at least 2 to 4 weeks before initiation of peels.

Precautions

Peeling must be cautiously performed for facial pigmentation in darker skins. Prolonged inflammation or excessive inflammation can stimulate the melanocyte and aggravate the pigmentation. Peeling should be avoided if there are open wounds and in patients who are careless about sun avoidance or postpeel care.

Peel Selection

The peeling agent should be chosen carefully according to the skin type of the patient and the depth of the pigmentation (Table 21.2). It is wiser to start with a lower concentration of peeling agent and gradually titrate upwards (Figures 21.1 to 21.4). Combining peels using lower concentrations is also safer. Though glycolic acid has been the most widely used peeling agent, it can cause PIH because the endpoint can be difficult to assess in very dark skins. Salicylic acid peel appears safer.[1] Khunger et al.[2] compared glycolic acid peels with 1% tretinoin as a peeling agent in melasma. The tretinoin peel was found to equally effective and better tolerated. Kalla et al.[3] compared 55 to 75% glycolic acid versus 10 to 15% trichloroacetic acid (TCA) peels in 100 patients with recalcitrant melasma. Response was quicker and better with TCA, but relapses were

Table 21.2: Selection of peeling agent according to the depth of the pigmentation

Depth of pigmentation	Peeling agent
Epidermal	Glycolic acid 30–50% applied for 1–3 minutes TCA 10–15% applied as 1 coat Jessner's solution 1–3 coats Salicylic acid 20% Mandelic acid 40% Phytic acid Lactic acid 50%
Mixed	Glycolic acid 70% applied for 3–30 minutes, depending on the type and thickness of the skin, till erythema appears TCA 25–35% Combination peels Glycolic acid 70% plus TCA 35%* Jessner's solution plus TCA 35%*

*In darker skins the concentration of TCA should be reduced to 25%

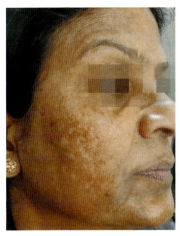

Fig. 21.1 Melasma in type V mature skin: start with low strength combination peel containing glycolic acid 20%, kojic acid, salicylic acid, citric acid, mandelic acid

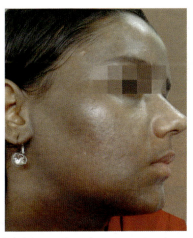

Fig. 21.2 Facial melanosis, dermal pigmentation due to lichen planus pigmentosus with sequential peel, 20% salicylic acid followed by 15% TCA. Start for 3 sessions at 2 week intervals. Follow with combination peel containing glycolic acid, kojic acid and citric acid

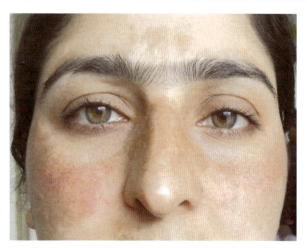

Fig. 21.3 Melasma in type III sensitive skin: salicylic acid 20% and with mandelic acid 20% in gel base

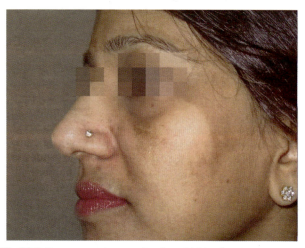

Fig. 21.4 Pigmentary demarcation lines with melasma: response to peels will be partial as PDL will not improve significantly

more common. Safoury et al.[4] compared the results of 15% TCA with 15% TCA followed by a modified Jessner's peel in a split face study of 20 patients with melasma with skin type II–IV. They found better results with the sequential peel as compared to TCA alone. Phytic acid has also found to be suitable for melasma in darker skins.[5] Another study confirmed the beneficial effect of peels with glycolic acid in melasma.[6]

Procedure

Informed consent and documentation with photographs are important prerequisites. Contact lenses should be removed. The face is cleaned and the hair is pulled back with a hair band or cap. The patient is either sitting or inclined at 45 degrees. The skin is cleaned with a prepeel cleanser and oily skin is degreased with acetone. The peeling agent of required strength is poured in a glass beaker and the neutralizing agent is kept ready. The agent is applied with a cotton tipped applicator on the entire face going along the cosmetic units. Begin from the forehead in an upward direction, then the right cheek, nose, left cheek and chin in that order. Feathering strokes are applied at the edges, to blend with surrounding skin and prevent demarcation lines.

It is important not to leave the room and closely watch for increasing redness, hot spots and epidermolysis. The peel is neutralized as required according to the peeling agent. The skin is gently dried with gauze and the patient is given ice packs till the burning subsides. The patient then applies a sunscreen, before leaving the clinic. A gel base peel or a retinol peel are leave on peels for 6 to 8 hours, hence are not neutralized.

Postpeel Care

Patients may feel tightness of the skin after a peel or may show frank desquamation, especially after the first peel (Figure 21.5). Following a retinol peel (yellow peel) exfoliation

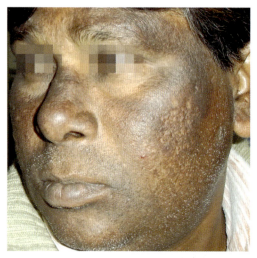

Fig. 21.5 Ochronosis due to self medicated prolonged use of hydroquinone: no response to chemical peels

or peeling of the skin occurs after 2 to 3 days and can last for 2 to 5 days. A non-comedogenic moisturizer may be used postpeel if the patient is uncomfortable. A mild soap or non-soap cleanser may be used. If there is crusting, topical antibacterial ointment should be used to prevent bacterial infection as older patients are much more prone to infection. Patients should be emphatically told to avoid peeling or scratching the skin. Superficial peels can be repeated every 2 weeks and medium depth peels may be repeated once a month.

Complications

The best way to avoid complications in patients with dark skins is to use prime the patient well, use combination peels and increase the strength of peeling agents gradually. A well primed skin will heal faster with fewer complications. Strict sun protection and good postpeel care are important. Post-inflammatory hyperpigmentation is most frequently seen, particularly if the patient has not been primed with skin lightening agents or there is excessive prolonged peeling combined with irritant dermatitis from topical retinoid or hydroquinone. Skin irritation, infection, flare up of herpes, and pigmentary abnormalities are complications that can occur following medium depth chemical peels. Excessive crusting, desquamation, inflammation and erythema can occur with all peels (Figure 21.5). Short course of mild topical steroid, like hydrocortisone can be prescribed for 2 to 4 days to tide over the inflammatory phase. In a review of treatment of melasma the most common adverse effects after peels were burning, dryness, skin irritation and erythema.[7]

Most of these were mild and transient. The skin returns to normal in superficial peels in 2 to 5 days and in 7 to 10 days in medium peels.

Key Points

√ Chemical peels are useful adjunctive procedures for facial pigmentation including melasma.

√ Thorough knowledge of various types is a must. Try and find the cause.

√ Topical therapy is very important. Combinations of treatment are required.

√ Chemical peels hasten response.

√ Counsel the patient before attempting chemical peels.

√ Adequate sun protection is a must.

√ Recurrences are common. Maintenance therapy is essential.

√ Lasers and IPL have changed the scenario, but the role of lasers is not yet fully established and equivocal in skin of color exposed to prolonged tropical sunlight.

√ Salicylic acid, mandelic acid, glycolic acid, Jessner's solution and TCA are peeling agents of choice used, singly or as combination peels.

References

1. Roberts WE. Chemical peeling in ethnic/dark skin. Dermatol Ther. 2004;17:196-205.
2. Khunger N, Sarkar R, Jain RK. Tretinoin peels versus glycolic acid peels in the treatment of melasma in dark skinned patients. Dermatol Surg. 2004;30(5):756-60.
3. Kalla G, Garg A, Kachhawa D. Chemical peeling—glycolic acid versus trichloroacetic acid in melasma. Indian J Dermatol Venereol. Leprol. 2001;67(2):82-4.
4. Safoury AS, Zaki NM, Nabarawy EAE, Farag EA. A study comparing chemical peeling using modified Jessner's solution and 15% trichloroacetic acid versus 15% trichloroacetic acid in the treatment of melasma. Ind J Derm. 2009;54:41-5.
5. Sarkar R, Bansal S, Garg VK. Chemical peels for melasma in dark-skinned patients. J Cutan Aesthet Surg. 2012;5(4):247-53.
6. Godse KV, Sakhia J. Triple combination and glycolic acid peels in melasma in Indian patients. J Cosmet Dermatol. 2011;10(1):68-9.
7. Rivas S, Pandya AG. Treatment of melasma with topical agents, peels and lasers: An evidence-based review. Am J Clin Dermatol. 2013;14(5):359-76.

22

Periocular Peels

Niti Khunger

- Common Problems in the Periocular Region
- Patient Assessment
- Counseling
- Priming and Preparation
- Precautions
- Peel Selection
- Procedure
- Postpeel Care
- Complications

Introduction

The eyes are one of the earliest and most prominent regions of the face to show signs of aging. Hence, treatment of the periocular area is vital to any holistic antiaging regimen. The periocular skin is thin, translucent and sensitive. Traditional techniques to rejuvenate the pericular complex like blepharoplasty are giving way to less invasive techniques such as botulinum toxin, chemical peels, fillers, autologous fat and lasers. Chemical peels are one of the most common noninvasive techniques to rejuvenate the skin.

Common Problems in the Periocular Region[1]

Dark circles: These are the most common problem in the periocular region, particularly in darker skins. The skin

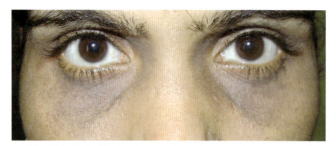

Fig. 22.1 Periorbital melanosis due to increased pigmentation

around the eyes appears hyperpigmented (Figure 22.1). They are caused by a combination of various factors. The possible causative factors include increased pigmentation, which is usually dermal, thin, translucent lower eyelid skin overlying the orbicularis oculi muscle, shadowing due to skin laxity, wrinkles and tear trough.[2] They can be genetic and be an extension of facial pigmentary demarcation lines (Figure 22.2). Rarely they may be due to facial acanthosis nigricans (Figure 22.3).

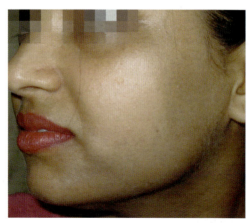

Fig. 22.2 Periocular pigmentation as an extension of facial pigmentary demarcation line type F

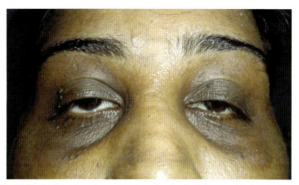

Fig. 22.3 Periocular pigmentation due to facial acanthosis nigricans with seborrheic keratosis in metabolic syndrome

Puffy eyes: The eyes appear puffy and swollen, a problem caused mainly by retention of fluid.

Under eye bags: This is accumulation of fat pads under the eyes, which appears as outpouchings in the lower eyelid (Figure 22.4).

Fine lines under eyes: The thin skin around the eyes loses its elasticity and becomes even thinner due to the breakdown of collagen during the aging process. Sun and environmental exposure can aggravate this (Figure 22.5).

Crow's feet: These are fine lines around the eyes at the lateral canthus caused due to expression like smiling and squinting (Figure 22.5).

Patient Assessment

The assessment of the patient should be objective and clearly written, taking into account the age, ethnic variations and social acceptability.

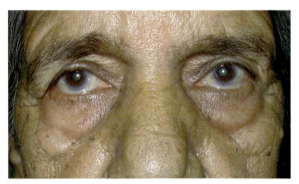

Fig. 22.4 Deep wrinkles and under eye bags due to herniation of fat

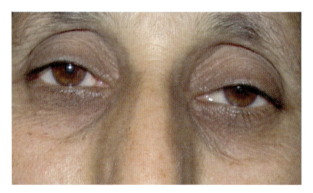

Fig. 22.5 Fine lines around the eye

First a holistic view of the periocular complex is undertaken. The skin color, texture, laxity and fine lines are assessed. The presence of fat herniation or eyebags, overhanging upper lids, ptosis, descent of the eyebrows, tear trough and malar bags are important conditions to be evaluated. It is crucial to then ask the patient which conditions are most bothersome as it may not be possible to address all the issues together. Often conditions what the physician feels require therapeutic intervention, may be acceptable to the patient and vice versa.

Chemical peels can improve skin color, texture and fine lines but cannot improve eyebags, tear trough or ptosis.

Counseling

Adequate counseling is the cornerstone for a successful skin rejuvenation program, particularly in the periorbital region. The patient must be clearly informed about the limitations of the improvement that can occur with chemical peels and expected outcomes must be lowered to avoid unsatisfied patients. The alternatives to treatment must be discussed and time taken for recovery of normal skin. Complications in particular pigmentary changes in darker skins must be spelt out and the importance of proper prepeel and postpeel care should be clearly explained. It should be emphasized that superficial peels are not one time procedures, but require multiple sessions and maintenance therapy as aging is also an ongoing process. Superficial chemical peeling is effective only for surface skin damage. The effects of aging in deeper tissues, such as fat herniation, deep wrinkles and drooping eyelids, must be addressed by other procedures.

Priming and Preparation

A priming regimen is essential before peeling, to enhance results and reduce risk of complications. Mature patients usually have dry thin skins; hence sunscreens with moisturizers are useful in the daytime. Topical retinoids have an additive effect as they improve skin texture, dyschromias and fine lines on prolonged usage. Retinol is better tolerated in the under eye area and is preferred. However, retinoid dermatitis is common in patients with mature dry and sensitive skin; hence it should be initially applied for short duration or alternate days, till tolerance develops. Low strength alpha hydroxy acids (AHAs) like glycolic acid 5 to 6% are also useful as they improve surface texture and also cause increase of collagen and ground substance in the dermis. Topical hypopigmenting agents are necessary in darker skins, to reduce the risk of postinflammatory hyperpigmentation (PIH). Undereye creams and vitamin C serums are also useful for priming and maintenance, in between and after the peels.

Precautions

Pigmentary changes are the main risk factors in darker skins, particularly on the eyelids. The thin skin of the eyelids is at an increased risk for scarring and color mismatch from the rest of the face. Care must be taken in doing deep peels, especially in skin types III–VI.

Peel Selection

One of the most common queries in a physician's mind is that can peels be safely performed in the delicate periocular region? Yes they can, provided a safe peel is selected and the technique is meticulously done.

Peels for the periocular areas must be carefully selected according to the pathology and skin type of the patient.[3] Superficial chemical peels are useful to improve hyperpigmentation, skin texture and fine lines. Young patients with minimal skin changes respond best to a series of peels. For older patients, chemical peels can be combined with other procedures like Botulinum toxin and fillers to achieve maximum benefit.

One of the safest peels for the periocular skin is low strength lactic acid as it has the properties of an alpha hydroxy acid along with a moisturizing effect. It has one of the largest molecules among AHAs, so the rate of penetration is much slower which results in less irritation to the skin. Thirty percent lactic acid can be initiated, gradually increasing the strength to 50%. It can also be used as a combination peel with citric acid, kojic acid, hydroquinone and salicylic acid. Lactic acid 15% combined with trichloroacetic acid (TCA) 3.75% in a proprietary formula was evaluated in 30 patients with dark circles. Fair to good improvement was seen in 93.3% of patients.[3] The effect of treatment lasted for 4 to 6 months. Complications included erythema, edema, frosting, dryness, and telangiectasias, which were mild and temporary.[4]

Polyhydroxy acids, including lactobionic acid and gluconolactone are chemically and functionally similar to alpha hydroxy acids. They are mild peeling agents and are incorporated in products for home use. They can be used in combination with other peeling agents for dry, sensitive skin of the eyelids. They do not cause irritation, stinging and burning as compared to AHAs and also have moisturizing, antioxidant and exfoliant properties.

Citric acid is a tricarboxylic acid, which is a powerful antioxidant and also has skin lightening properties. It is used in a concentration of 10 to 50% as a home peeling agent and 20 to 70% as an office procedure.

Retinol peels are particularly useful for dark circles that are caused by a combination of hyperpigmentation and aging skin as seen in mature patients. But they can cause a lot of exfoliation and have to be handled carefully in the postpeel period.

Trichloroacetic acid peels have been used singly or in combination and they are safe in a concentration of 10 to 15%, even in dark skins.

Arginine has also been used as a peeling agent in combination with lactic acid. But it is a very mild peeling agent and has not shown a significant response in the author's experience. It may be useful only in young patients with mild changes.

Deep peels such as phenol peels are effective as single procedures and also have a significant skin tightening effect. Various formulae for phenol peels have been used but for the periocular area Hetter's peel[5] and Litton's phenol peel[6] (phenol, 44 mL; distilled water, 44 mL; and croton oil, 1 mL; creating a phenol concentration of 48%) are popular over the Baker-Gordon peel formula. At these concentrations, the phenol penetrates up to the reticular dermis. This causes significant skin tightening and hypopigmentation, which can be prolonged in darker skins. Hence, they should preferably be performed only in skin type I–III and by experienced physicians as there is a very low margin of safety in such peels.

Procedure

Photodocumentation and informed consent is essential before starting the peels. The peel should be carried out with the patient sitting comfortably with a head rest or lying down with the head elevated to 45°.

- A syringe containing saline should be kept ready before starting the procedure, in case the peeling agent enters the eye.
- The skin is prepared as for all peel procedures. But prepeel cleansing should be gentle using a prepeel cleanser rather than degreasing with acetone. The delicate skin of the eyelids should be carefully handled to avoid minor abrasions which can increase the peel depth and cause PIH and even scarring.
- The inner and outer canthi should be protected with vaseline. If peeling the upper eyelid the lash margin should be protected with vaseline. For the lower eyelid a very thin layer of vaseline should be applied near the lash margin to prevent the peel from entering the eye. Alternatively neomycin eye ointment can be applied just within the eye margin.
- In my opinion, the eye should be peeled one at a time to maintain control of the spread of the peeling agent. The skin is stretched and the peel is gently applied with a cotton

bud. The skin should be kept stretched till the peeling is completed. The peel is then cleansed off and then the other eye is peeled. This reduces the risk of the peel gathering in the tear trough area or entering the eye. One should never leave the room when doing a periocular peel, nor entrust the assistant.

- After the peel, a moisturizer with sunscreen is applied.

Postpeel Care

The skin may feel tight after the procedure and may appear wrinkled because of desquamation. This can be treated by repeated application of moisturizers. If there is excessive inflammation edema can occur because of the lax skin. A short course of oral steroids prednisolone 20 mg per day for 3 to 5 days is sufficient along with ice compresses. Superficial peels can be repeated every 2 weeks, medium depth peels may be repeated after 6 to 9 months, while deep peels should not be repeated before one year.

Complications

It is essential to use utmost care in the periocular region as complications can occur more commonly in this area as compared to other regions. The best way to avoid complications is to initially use milder peels and gradually increase the strength. Combination peels or combinant procedures are preferred as they provide maximum effect with minimal risks. Skin irritation, edema, crusting, prolonged erythema, postinflammatory hyperpigmentation can occur. Infection and scarring with ectropion may occur following deep peels. Frequent application of moisturizers, topical steroid cream like hydrocortisone 1% are used to reduce side effects. The skin returns to normal in superficial peels in 2 to 5 days and in 7 to 10 days in medium depth peels.

COMBINATION PROCEDURES

Peels can be combined with botulinum toxin for the crows feet, fillers for the tear trough, fractional ablative or nonablative lasers or fractional radiofrequency for skin tightening. Chemical peels can also be combined with blepharoplasty to improve surface texture.

Conclusion

Chemical peels are a useful armamentarium in the modalities for rejuvenation. They are versatile, offer significant benefit with minimum downtime. The choice of peeling agents can be varied according to skin type, offering a good safety profile in experienced hands. They are cost effective with few complications. They are safe in the periocular region provided they are done carefully.

Key Points

√ Chemical peeling in the periocular area is a minimally invasive and effective procedure in experienced hands.
√ It promotes dermal collagen along with improving surface texture, mild wrinkling and also has a skin tightening effect.
√ Thus, it can be useful for dark circles, mild wrinkles and skin tightening on repeated applications.
√ Glycolic acid, lactic acid, retinol peels are commonly used in the periocular area.
√ Chemical peeling can also be combined with other techniques such as botulinum toxin, fillers and blepharoplasty for an additive effect.
√ Attention should also be paid to lifestyle changes, proper nutrition and sleep and sun protection.

References

1. Nanda S, Bansal S. Upper face rejuvenation using botulinum toxin and hyaluronic acid fillers. Indian J Dermatol Venereol Leprol. 2013;79:32-40

2. Roh MR, Chung KY. Infraorbital dark circles: definition, causes and treatment options. Dermatol Surg. 2009;35:1163-71.

3. Cantisano-Zilkha. An ophthalmologist's guide to chemical Peels. Ophthalmol Clin N Am. 2005;18:227-35.

4. Vavouli C, Katsambas A, Gregoriou S, Teodor A, Salavastru C, Alexandru A, et al. Chemical peeling with trichloroacetic acid and lactic acid for infraorbital dark circles. J Cosmet Dermatol. 2013;12:204-9.

5. Hetter GP. An examination of the phenol-croton oil peel: part IV. Face peel results with different concentrations of phenol and croton oil. Plast Reconstr Surg. 2000;105(3):1081-3.

6. Epstein JS. Management of infraorbital dark circles a significant cosmetic concern. Arch Facial Plast Surg. 1999;1:303-7.

23

Complications

Niti Khunger

- Evaluating Patients at Risk
- Basic Precautions
- Avoiding Complications
- Managing Complications

Introduction

The occurrence of complications is inherent in every procedure, and every physician performing chemical peels must have adequate knowledge about early detection, management and prevention of complications. A well-informed and cooperative patient is an asset to the physician in minimizing risks of adverse effects. An experienced practitioner develops individual guidelines, evolved over a period of time, that help in performing safe procedures in different types of skins. This chapter mainly concentrates on practices that minimize risks of complications in ethnic darker skin types.

Evaluating Patients at Risk

There are a certain group of patients that are at a higher risk of complications. It is important to identify these individuals, so that adverse events can be anticipated and treated at the earliest.

- Skin types III-VI are at a higher risk of postinflammatory hyperpigmentation (PIH)
- Patients with thin, dry and delicate skin with a reddish hue
- Patients with outdoor occupations
- History of sunburn and PIH
- Patients on photosensitizing drugs
- Patients with sensitive skin or history of atopic dermatitis
- Uncooperative, fussy, obsessed, unrealistic, difficult-to-please, doctor-shopping patients.

Basic Precautions

It is important to remember that results cannot be guaranteed and every patient is at potential risk of complications. The physician should take all precautions to avoid complications and communicate to the patient early warning signs of adverse events. Most complications can be minimized, when detected early and treated promptly.

- At the first visit take all relevant history and assess the patient for potential complications like heavy sun exposure, sensitive skin, PIH, keloids, poor wound healing and photosensitizing applications and medications. Ask specifically about over-the-counter (OTC) drugs and herbal preparations. Patients applying potent topical steroids develop thin skins and are at increased risk for complications.
- Educate the patient about early warning signs like prolonged erythema, PIH, crusting, etc.
- Give clear unambiguous instructions to the patient and emphasize the importance of following instructions carefully.
- Emphasize that superficial chemical peeling is a procedure requiring repeated applications, where results take a longer time to show and, maintenance peels are required. Superficial peels are safer, with minimal downtime but will not help in deeper lesions.
- Do not use too many peels of different manufacturers. Peels from different sources, even with the same labeled

concentrations can have varying results. It is better to be familiar with fewer peels on a regular basis.

- When trying out a new peel, or peeling an apprehensive patient, preferably do a test peel on the preauricular area, or a small area on the lesion on the forehead or temple area, rather than a full face peel.
- Start with the lowest concentration and gradually titrate upwards.
- Initially, if results are unsatisfactory, it is better to combine different agents at lower concentrations, rather than use a high concentration of a single peeling agent.
- Tell patients to avoid scrubs and any other procedure, immediately before peels as it can lead to uneven peeling. It has been observed that bleaching of the face with ammonia (commonly done in dark skin patients) within one week after a peel can lead to irritant dermatitis (personal observation).
- Take good and adequate photographs, so it is easier to monitor progress.

Avoiding Complications[1,2]

PREPEEL

- Identify patients at risk by a detailed history and examination and take adequate steps like priming the skin for 2 to 4 weeks prior to the peel.
- Counsel the patient and discuss expected results, need for applying topical treatment after peels for maintenance and preventing complications.

DURING THE PEEL

- Selection of the right peel at the right concentration. It is better to underpeel than overpeel in the initial stages. Keep the selected peel on the table and remove the others.
- Check the label of the peel and the expiry date (Figures 23.1A and B). The potency of glycolic acid decreases

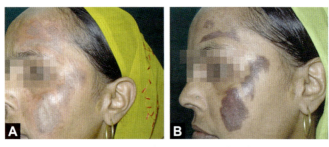

Figs 23.1A and B Complication due to improper labeling application of 35% TCA instead of 35% GA. Persistent hyperpigmentation for 6 months

with time. Trichloroacetic acid (TCA) lasts for approximately 6 months. The potency of salicylic acid peels and all peels in alcoholic solution can become more potent with time due to evaporation of alcohol.

- Do not use the peeling agent directly from the bottle. Crystals may be present which can adhere to the cotton tip and increase concentration.
- Keep the neutralizing agent ready in case termination of the peel is required before the scheduled time.
- Vigorous scrubbing should be avoided as it can lead to patchy deeper peels than required.
- Keep a syringe filled with saline ready, in case of accidental spillage in the eye. If TCA or glycolic acid (GA) enters the eye flood it with normal saline. For phenolic compounds, the eye should be flooded with mineral oil.
- Do not pass the peel bottle or swab over the eye, while applying the peel.
- *Periocular peels:* When applying a peel near the eyes, keep a dry applicator ready to mop up tears. If there is tearing of the eyes the peel can trickle up or down. Stretch the wrinkles near the eyes and then apply the peel and keep on holding till there is frosting or burning has stopped. Watch out for hot spots and epidermolysis neutralize the peel immediately (Figure 23.2).

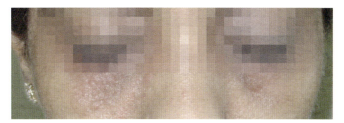

Fig. 23.2 Periorbital epidermolysis with 70% glycolic acid

POSTPEEL

- Topical antibiotic ointment and moisturizers postpeel enhance wound healing. Povidone-iodine, tretinoin and steroids delay wound healing and should be avoided till re-epithelialization occurs.
- Sun exposure should be avoided, especially in dark skin patients and in those with pigmentary disorders.

Managing Complications[1-9] (Tables 23.1 to 23.3)

Serious complications are rare with superficial peels. Since these peels are light peels, results are not dramatic and quick. Hence, unmet expectations are the most common cause of complications in these patients.

EDEMA

Edema can occur within 24 to 72 hours of chemical peeling. It is uncommon in superficial peels, but can be seen in patients with thin atrophic dry skin and in the periocular area. Application of ice is helpful and it usually subsides spontaneously. In severe cases, a short course of systemic steroids may be given.

Table 23.1: Complications of superficial peels

- Edema
- Pain and burning
- Persistent erythema
- *Pruritus*
- Bacterial infection
- Herpetic infection
- Candidal infection
- Hyperpigmentation
- Hypopigmentation
- Demarcation lines
- Ocular complications
  Acneiform eruptions
- Allergic reactions
  Scarring
- Toxicity
- Laryngeal edema

Table 23.2: Complications of medium and deep peels

- Persistent erythema
- Hyperpigmentation
- Hypopigmentation
- Scarring
- Infection
- Toxicity
- Milia
- Delayed healing
- Textural changes

Table 23.3: Complications of peels and their management

Mild	Management	Moderate	Management	Severe	Management
Edema	Ice application Systemic steroids	Hyper-pigmentation	Peel holiday for 4 weeks Sunscreens Skin lightening agents	Hypo to depigmen-tation	Occurs due to phenol peels in darker skins Management very difficult Topical trimethylpsoralen lotion NB UVB therapy
Transient erythema	Sunscreens Topical steroids	Acneiform eruptions	Oral antibiotics Topical antibiotics Benzoyl peroxide 2.5% cream base	Atrophic scarring	Microneedling Nonablative fractional lasers Excision of scars
Irritation	Moisturizers Mild topical steroids	Persistent erythema	Sunscreens Potent topical steroids for short duration Intralesional steroids Pulsed dye laser if no response	Hypertrophic scarring	Intralesional steroids Massage Pulsed dye laser

Contd...

Contd...

Mild	Management	Moderate	Management	Severe	Management
Pruritus	Mild topical steroids Oral antihistamines Look for contact dermatitis	Contact dermatitis	Stop irritant medications Oral antihistamines Topical steroids Systemic steroids	Line of demarcation	
Scaling	Moisturizers Topical steroids Stop topical retinoids and glycolic acid as home regimen	Excessive crusting	Topical and systemic antibiotics	Spillage in the eye Ectropion	
Excessive desquamation	Moisturizers Topical steroids	Prolonged scaling	Stop further peels till skin is normal Moisturizers		
Feeling of heat	Sign of overpeeling Stop peeling Give a peel holiday for 4–8 weeks	Herpes infection Pain and burning Sensitive skin Dissatisfied patient	Acyclovir and antibiotics Sign of overpeeling—stop peeling Change modality of treatment		

BLISTERING

Epidermolysis, vesiculation and blistering can occur, particularly with alpha hydroxy acid (AHA) due to deeper peels. It is more common in younger patients and around the eyes, with loose periorbital skin (Figure 23.2).

PAIN AND BURNING

This is common during the peel, but in patients with sensitive skin can persist up to 2 to 5 days after the peel, till complete re-epithelialization. Using topical retinoid or glycolic acid immediately after peels and prolonged sun exposure can also lead to persistent burning. Application of bland emollients and sunscreens are effective, however, in some patients, sunscreens can also cause irritation. Topical calamine lotion is soothing and in severe cases, topical steroids like hydrocortisone or fluticasone may be required.

PERSISTENT ERYTHEMA

Though erythema can be seen after all peels, it is not common in superficial peels. Generally, erythema fades in 3 to 5 days, after superficial peels, 15 to 30 days after medium peels and 60 to 90 days after deep peels. However, prolonged erythema may be a sign of inadvertent deeper peeling and impending scarring. It should be treated with potent topical steroids for 2 to 5 days, and with intralesional steroids, if there is no response (Figure 23.3).

PRURITUS

Pruritus following re-epithelialization can occur after superficial peels, though it is more common after medium and deep peels. When it occurs with the development of papules, pustules and erythema, it may be due to a contact dermatitis to a topical application. It is very important to recognize this and

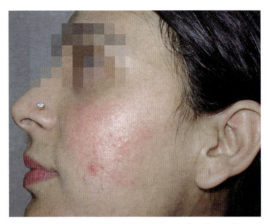

Fig. 23.3 Persistent erythema due to glycolic acid 70%

treat as soon as possible, as a delay in treatment can cause PIH in darker skins, worsening the outcome of the peel. Hence, it is preferable that no new topical agents should be introduced in the maintenance regime after a peel to avoid this complication.

INFECTIONS

Infections are uncommon with superficial peels, but can occur in hot humid climates with excessive sweating. Impetigo and folliculitis can occur due to staphylococci and should be appropriately treated with cloxacillin or amoxycillin-clavulanic acid combination. *Streptococcus* and *Pseudomonas* infections can also occur and should be treated with appropriate antibiotics. Topical wound care is important. Wound should be cleaned 3 to 4 times a day with potassium permanganate soaks and topical mupirocin ointment for Gram positive organisms should be used.

Candidal infection in the form of superficial pustules can occur in patients who are immunocompromised, applying prolonged topical steroids and in diabetics and patients with oral thrush. They should be treated with topical clotrimazole 1% and systemic antifungals such as fluconazole 50 mg or ketoconazole 200 mg per day.

Herpetic infection can be precipitated following peels, though it is more common with medium and deep peels as compared to superficial peels. The presence of herpetic infection developing after a peel can cause scarring. It presents as sudden appearance of grouped erosions, associated with pain. Hence prophylactic antiviral such as acyclovir 200 mg, 5 times a day or valaciclovir 1 gm, 3 times a day should be given, beginning 2 days prior to the peel and continued for 10 to 14 days after peeling till re-epithelialization occurs. It should be given to all patients with active lesions or history of herpes simplex, undergoing medium and deep peels and in patients with active herpetic lesions undergoing superficial peels.

HYPERPIGMENTATION

Hyperpigmentation is very common, in patients with skin types III to VI undergoing superficial or medium peels. It can occur any time after the peel and can be persistent, if inadequately treated. Hence it is important to educate the patient about avoiding sun exposure and use of broad spectrum sunscreens before and indefinitely after the peels. Hyperpigmentation can also occur in patients using photosensitizing drugs such as NSAIDs, oral contraceptives, etc. Hyperpigmentation can also occur in type I to II skins following intense sun exposure and tanning or use of photosensitizing agents.

Priming the patient with suitable topical hypopigmenting agents such as hydroquinone, kojic acid, arbutin, etc. is an important part of the peeling regimen and should be strictly enforced in the post peel period. When hyperpigmentation occurs, triple combinations of hydroquinone, tretinoin and steroids are useful and are restarted as soon as re-epithelialization is complete (Figures 23.4A and B).

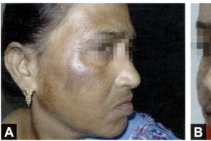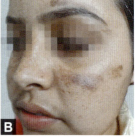

Figs 23.4A and B (A) Persistent hyperpigmentation due to 15% TCA; (B) PIH following a sequential peel, 20% salicylic acid followed by 15% TCA

HYPOPIGMENTATION

A lighter complexion is often seen after peeling and is much sought after by darker skins. This effect is transient in superficial peels due to sloughing off of the epidermis and removal of excess melanin. In medium peels, with removal of the basal layer, the hypopigmentation can be more prolonged, till melanocytes migrate from the surrounding skin and adnexae. In darker skins this hypopigmentation can be followed by PIH, due to over activity of the melanocytes, hence medium peels are done with great caution in darker individuals. In deep peels, permanent hypopigmentation is common, which is not noticeable in fair type I and II skins, but can have disastrous consequences in darker skins. Hence deep peels are better avoided in darker skin types. Phenol in addition has a direct toxic effect on the melanocytes and can cause a permanent hypopigmentation with a peculiar alabaster look. If hypopigmentation is very noticeable the untreated areas of the face and neck should be peeled to avoid lines of demarcation (Figure 23.5).

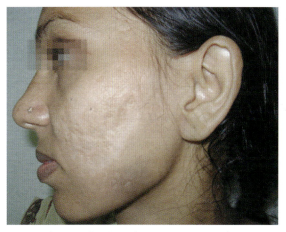

Fig. 23.5 Persistent hypopigmentation due to medium depth peeling with TCA

LINES OF DEMARCATION

These are lines of pigmentary change at the junction of peeled and unpeeled areas. They are common in all skin types and more common in darker skins and medium and deep peels. The periocular, perioral and jaw line are common sites of predilection. To avoid this, peeling agent with a lower concentration should be feathered at the edges to merge with the surrounding normal skin.

DELAYED HEALING

Delayed healing can occur due to infection, irritation, premature peeling, in patients undergone previous facial surgery, radiation or immunocompromised states. Aggressive wound care management is important to prevent infection and scarring. Topical mupirocin ointment along with systemic antibiotics with good coverage of staphylococci should be given till re-epithelialization is complete.

OCULAR INJURIES[7]

All peeling agents can cause damage to the eyes in case of accidental spillage. Care must be taken particularly when peeling the periorbital area and a dry swab stick must be kept ready to absorb any tears. The peeling agent must not be passed across the eye. In case of accidental spillage, the eyes should be flushed copiously with normal saline to prevent corneal damage.

In case of phenol peels, the eye must be flushed with mineral oil, instead of saline.

ACNEIFORM ERUPTIONS

Acneiform eruptions can occur in patients who are prone to developing acne. It usually results from the occlusive effects of ointments applied after a peel and is more common with glycolic acid peels. It presents as erythematous tender nodules occurring after a peel. They are treated with systemic antibiotics and topical antibiotic creams in cream base, rather than gel base, which can act as an irritant. They usually resolve in 7 to 10 days after treatment.

ALLERGIC REACTIONS

Allergic reactions to chemical peels are rare. Resorcinol has a higher incidence of allergic reactions, while cholinergic urticaria has been reported following TCA peels. Allergic reactions to the topical reagents used in the maintenance phase are commoner, particularly due to sunscreens, hydroquinone and tretinoin. Hence these should be used with care and stopped at the first sign of allergy, to avoid PIH.

SCARRING

Scarring is very uncommon, after superficial peels, unless peeling has been uneven and deeper in localized areas. It is more common with deeper peels, particularly in patients who have premature peeling or infection or reactions during the peel. Sites with a predilection for scarring are the temple area, mandibular area upper lips and the chin. Scars can be flat hypopigmented and shiny with loss of texture or depressed atrophic with sharp demarcation. Thickened, hypertrophic keloidal scarring can occur in prone individuals with medium peels, especially over the jaw area. In severe cases, there can be ectropion or eclabion. Atypical hypertrophic stellate scars in the mid cheek area have been reported in patients undergoing, resurfacing procedures, who were on isotretinoin for 2 to 3 years before the procedure. This may be due to decreased collagenase or impaired collagen remodeling due to isotretinoin. However it is extremely rare and many reports show that it does not always occur. Anyway, it is prudent to avoid medium and deep peels for 6 months in patients who have had long term isotretinoin.

Once scarring begins to develop, due to any cause, it must be treated aggressively. Flat atrophic scars are difficult to treat, while hypertrophic scars should be treated with potent topical steroids, clobetasol proprionate for 2 weeks followed by mometasone till erythema and induration disappear. The pulsed dye laser may also be useful in treating incipient scarring and reducing erythema.

TOXICITY

TCA and glycolic acid are not absorbed systemically; hence systemic toxicity is not reported. Salicylic acid can be absorbed after application over large areas and cause salicylism. Tinnitus, nausea, vomiting, gastrointestinal irritation are the presenting features. This can be potentiated if the patient also ingests aspirin.

COMPLICATIONS OF MEDIUM AND DEEP PEELS

All the above complications of superficial peels can occur with medium and deep peels and are in fact much more common as compared to superficial peels.

Pigmentary changes are the most common, particularly in darker skin patients. Hyperpigmentation is common, almost inevitable, with medium peels, while permanent hypopigmentation or depigmentation can occur with deep phenol peels in ethnic dark skins. Hence these peels are relatively contraindicated in darker type III to VI skins (see Figure 23.5).

Scarring can occur with medium depth and deep peels. Patients with a history of poor wound healing, keloid formation and who develop postpeel infection are more prone to developing scarring. Peeling in nonfacial areas such as neck, dorsal of hands and chest that do not have sufficient adnexae to re-epithelize are more prone to scarring. Patients on isotretinoin have been reported to show abnormal scarring, following deep peels. This is still controversial, but it is better to wait for at least 6 months after stopping isotretinoin before attempting deep chemical peels. Early signs of scarring include persistent erythema and pruritis. Potent topical steroids should be used without delay. If wounds have not re-epithelized after 2 weeks, they have a potential for scarring and should be adequately treated with antibiotics and biological dressings along with good wound care. Herpetic infections can occur in susceptible patients and lead to scarring. Hence all patients undergoing medium or deep peels should be given prophylactic acyclovir or valacyclovir 500 mg bd beginning 2 days before the peel and continued for 2 weeks after the peel, till complete re-epithelialization.

ECTROPION

Ectropion can develop in a phenol peel, when applied in the periocular area. It is more common in patients who have undergone blepharoplasties previously.

Milia may occur 2 to 3 weeks after re-epithelialization, following medium and deep peels. Occlusive ointments must be avoided and they frequently show spontaneous resolution. If the patient demands, extraction or light electrodessication may be done.

TEXTURAL CHANGES

Textural changes of the skin can occur due to uneven depths of the peeling. This can be due to improper priming, skin preparation or faulty technique. Retinoid dermatitis and reactions due to topical agents prior to peeling can result in deeper penetration of the peel. Patients must be asked to stop retinoids and AHA products 2 to 5 days before the peel. During skin preparation, degreasing must be uniform and while application of the peel, the peeling agent must be applied uniformly. Hence it is easier to apply peeling agents that cause visible frosting such as TCA, salicylic acid, resorcinol and tretinoin.

TOXICITY

Resorcinol can produce toxicity, if applied in excess. It presents with diarrhea, vomiting, dizziness, drowsiness, severe headache, bradycardia, dyspnea and paralysis. The best way to avoid resorcinism is to restrict the area of application or limit the concentration of resorcinol.

Phenol can cause toxicity if applied over large areas over a short period or under-occlusion. The most common systemic adverse effect is cardiotoxicity, presenting in the form of arrhythmias. To avoid this complication, cardiac status must be monitored and intravenous hydration be given. If arrhythmia develops, the peel must be stopped and IV lignocaine should be administered. Since phenol is metabolized in the liver and excreted by the kidney, it should not be used in patients with hepatorenal disease.

DRUG INTERACTIONS

Lignocaine with adrenaline should be used with caution in patients with tachycardia. Drugs which can cause arrhythmias such as diuretics, monoamine oxidase (MAO) inhibitors, phenothiazine and tricyclic antidepressants should be stopped 1 to 2 weeks before using lignocaine with adrenaline. Heavy smokers should preferably be avoided, while doing deep phenol peels, due to the risk of delayed healing and scarring.

Some rare complications reported one airway compromise after alpha hydroxy facial peels.[10]

Conclusion

Though peels can cause complications, they are uncommon in well-trained hands. Pigmentary changes are the most common and most persistent complications seen, especially in darker ethnic skins. Superficial peels cause hyperpigmentation and deeper peels cause hypopigmentation. Adequate patient counseling and education and performing peels carefully with all basic precautions are the two main factors in minimizing the risks of chemical peels.

References

1. Duffy DM. Avoiding complications with chemical peels. In: Rubin MG (Ed): Chemical peels. Procedures in cosmetic dermatology. Elsevier Inc., 2006.pp.137-70.
2. Fanous N. A new patient classification for laser resurfacing and peels: Predicting responses, risks and results. Aesthetic Plast Surg. 2002;26(2):99-104.

3. Rubin MG. Complications. In: Manual of chemical peel. Manual of chemical peels—superficial and medium depth. 1st edn. Philadelphia. JB Lippincot Co; 1995.pp.130-53.

4. Brody HJ. Complications of chemical peels. Chemical peeling and resurfacing. 2nd edn. Mosby Year Book Inc; 1997.pp.162-94.

5. Coleman KM, Coleman WP. Complications of chemical peeling. In: Rubin MG (Ed): Chemical peels. Procedures in cosmetic dermatology. Elsevier Inc; 2006.pp.171-83.

6. Resnik SS, Resnik BI. Complications of chemical peeling. Dermatol Clin. 1995;13(2):309-12. Review.

7. Landau M. Cardiac complications in deep chemical peels. Dermatol Surg. 2007;33(2):190-3; discussion 193.

8. Fung JF, Sengelmann RD, Kenneally CZ. Chemical injury to the eye from trichloroacetic acid. Dermatol Surg. 2002;28(7):609-10; discussion 610.

9. Grimes PE. The safety and efficacy of salicylic acid chemical peels in darker racial-ethnic groups. J Dermatol Surg. 1999;25:18-22.

10. Ghadishah D, Gorchynski J. Airway compromise after routine alpha-hydroxy facial peel administration. J Emerg Med. 2002;22(4):353-5.

24

Interesting Case Studies

Niti Khunger, Shenaz Arsiwala, Jaishree Sharad

Chemical peeling has become popular in today's milieu of aesthetics because it is simple to perform, can be done as an office procedure, requires no equipment or maintenance, has virtually no downtime and is cost effective. Acne, pigmentation and skin rejuvenation form the bulk of an aesthetic practice, particularly, in ethnic skins and chemicals peels can address all these issues. The advent of safe and versatile peeling agents has further enhanced the utility of peels. In this chapter, interesting cases are discussed emphasizing on the choice of peels that can be utilized to give optimum results.

Case 1

Niti Khunger

PROBLEM

- Resistant extensive inflammatory adult acne Grade 3, with PIH.
- Type IV thick oily skin (Figures 24.1A to D).

SOLUTION

Priming: Start systemic antibiotic azithromycin. Doxycycline can cause phototoxicity and aggravate pigmentation. Prime the skin with sunscreen gel base in the morning, hydroquinone 5% in the evening and clindamycin in combination with 0.025% tretinoin for 1 hour in the evening for 2 weeks.

Peeling: After 2 weeks chemical peel with salicylic acid 20% every 2 weeks for 4 to 6 weeks.

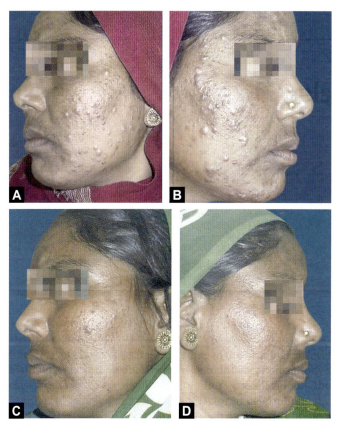

Figs 24.1A to D (A and B) Extensive inflammatory acne, type IV thick oily skin; (C and D) Salicylic acid 20% peels

Case 2

Niti Khunger

PROBLEM

- Inflammatory acne, with few pustules, postacne erythema and inflammatory scars
- Type IV thin sensitive skin.

SOLUTION

Priming: Start antibiotics, doxycycline or azithromycin. Prime the skin with physical sunscreen lotion containing zinc oxide in the morning, clindamycin in combination with adapalene for 1 hour in the evening for 2 weeks.

Peeling: After 2 weeks chemical peel with mandelic acid 40% every week for 2 weeks. After 2 weeks, add sequential peel, 20% salicylic acid for 10 minutes followed by mandelic acid or combination peel salicylic-mandelic acid, every 2 weeks. Alternatively use lactic acid peels (Figures 24.2A to D).

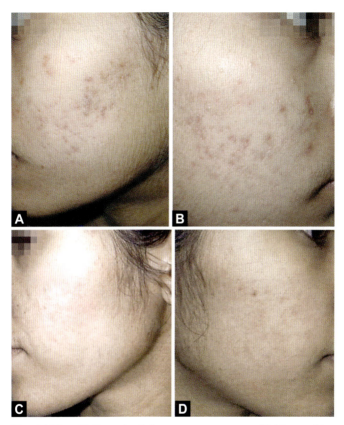

Figs 24.2A to D Extensive inflammatory acne, type IV thin sensitive skin, mandelic acid and salicylic acid peels: (A and B) Before treatment; (C and D) After treatment

Case 3

Niti Khunger

PROBLEM

- Resistant acne with melasma
- Type V skin, with tendency to postinflammatory hyperpigmentation.

SOLUTION

Priming: Sunscreen with hydroquinone in the day. Glycolic acid 10% with hydroquinone 4% in the evening for 1 to 2 hours. Tretinoin 0.025% in the night for 4 weeks. Avoid using triple combinations with steroid, which can aggravate acne.

Peeling: Sequential peel salicylic acid peel 20%, wash after 10 minutes followed by mandelic acid 40% till acne improves. Then add sequential peel glycolic acid 35% for 3 minutes, wash apply salicylic acid 20 to 40%. Increase strength of glycolic acid gradually. If no response add combination peel, kojic acid with glycolic acid (Figures 24.3A to D).

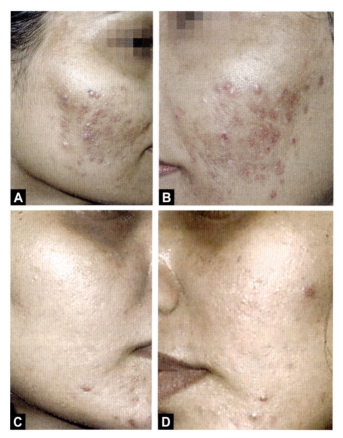

Figs 24.3A to D Sequential peels salicylic acid followed by mandelic acid, subsequently glycolic acid peels: (A and B) Before treatment; (C and D) After treatment

Case 4

Niti Khunger

PROBLEM

- Cystic acne with hypertrophic scars
- Type V skin.

SOLUTION

Priming: Start azithromycin 500 mg on three consecutive days a week for 4 weeks along with NSAID anti-inflammatory ibuprofen to reduce inflammation. Drain the cysts, evacuate the contents and destroy the walls by phenolization. Give intralesional triamcinolone acetonide 5 mg/mL to prevent and reduce hypertrophic scarring. Topical clindamycin gel in the morning and tretinoin 0.0255 in the evening.

Peeling: Follow-up with comedone extraction and salicylic acid peels 20%, every 2 weeks. Salicylic acid is comedolytic and anti-inflammatory (Figures 24.4A to C).

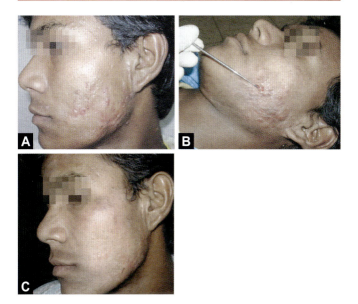

Figs 24.4A to C Cystic acne with hypertrophic scars, type V skin, evacuate the cysts, phenolize, ILS. Followed by comedone extraction and salicylic acid peels

Case 5

Niti Khunger

PROBLEM

- Superficial acne scars, sensitive skin unable to tolerate glycolic acid products, mild melasma
- Type IV skin.

SOLUTION

Priming: Sunscreen containing physical blocker only, zinc oxide 15% in the morning. Hypopigmenting cream containing kojic acid 2% and vitamin C in the evening. Adapalene 1% gel for 1 hour twice a week.

Peeling: Sequential peels with salicylic acid peels 20%, washed after 10 minutes followed by mandelic acid 40% left overnight. Repeated every 2 weeks for 4 peels (Figures 24.5A to D).

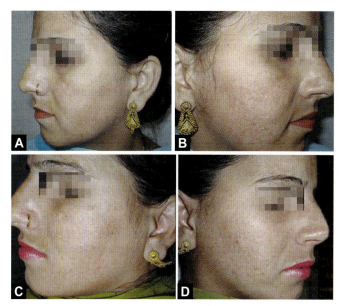

Figs 24.5A to D Superficial acne scars with melasma in sensitive skin, Sequential peels with salicylic acid followed by mandelic acid: (A and B) Before treatment; (C and D) After treatment

Case 6

Niti Khunger

PROBLEM

- Postacne scars
- Type IV skin.

SOLUTION

Priming: Patient was first primed with sunscreen in the day and hydroquinone and tretinoin in the night for 4 weeks.

Peeling: Manual dermasanding was done with autoclaved sandpaper, P220, till pinpoint bleeding, followed by TCA 15%. Punch excision and suturing of deep scars was done using appropriate size punch. Procedure was repeated after 6 weeks (Figures 24.6A to D).

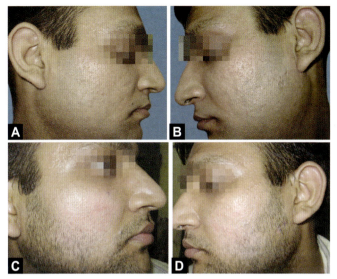

Figs 24.6A to D Post acne scars treated with manual dermasanding and 15% TCA: (A and B) Before treatment; (C and D) After treatment

Case 7

Niti Khunger

PROBLEM

- Icepick scars
- Type V skin with tendency to PIH and herpes simplex.

SOLUTION

Priming: Patient was primed with hydroquinone 4% along with sun protection and sunscreens in the day. Glycolic acid 10% with kojic acid 2% alternated with tretinoin 0.025% in the night for 4 weeks. Herpes simplex was treated with famciclovir 250 mg tid for 5 days.

Peeling: Icepick scars were treated with CROSS technique using 100% TCA. Acyclovir 400 mg bd was given for 10 days till complete healing. CROSS technique was repeated after 1 month (Figures 24.7A to F).

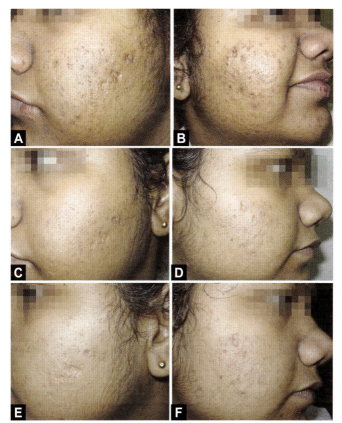

Figs 24.7A to F Icepick scars, type V skin with tendency to PIH, treated with CROSS technique 100% TCA: (A and B) Before treatment; (C and D) After 1 session of CROSS technique; (E and F) After 2 sessions of CROSS technique

Case 8

Niti Khunger

PROBLEM

- Dermal pigmentation—pigmented cosmetic dermatitis, resistant to topical treatment
- Type V skin.

SOLUTION

Priming: Priming the skin with sunscreen in combination with hydroquinone 4% in the morning, triple combination of hydroquinone 2%, tretinoin 0.025% and mometasone 0.1% at night.

Peeling: Patient was treated with sequential peels. Glycolic acid 70% for 3 to 5 minutes followed by salicylic acid 30% were given at 2 weekly intervals for 6 months. There was a plateau in the response, subsequently combination peels were added glycolic acid, kojic acid and hydroquinone weekly for 2 months. (Glyco K) (Figures 24.8A to F).

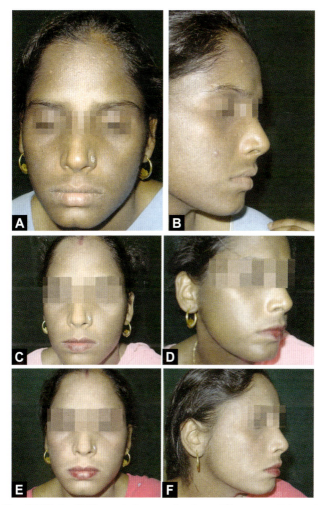

Figs 24.8A to F Pigmented cosmetic dermatitis, sequential peels, glycolic acid followed by salicylic acid: (A and B) Before treatment; (C and D) After 2 peels; (E and F) After 20 peels

Case 9

Niti Khunger

PROBLEM

Macular amyloidosis on the back.

SOLUTION

Priming: Adequate priming with potent topical steroid clobetasol twice a day and triple combination twice a day.

Peeling: 20% salicylic acid peels at 2 week intervals were done for 4 peels. This helps in decreasing superficial pigment and allows deeper penetration of hypopigmenting agents like hydroquinone. There was about 20% improvement. Then combination peel of glycolic acid, kojic acid and hydroquinone was done weekly for 4 weeks. Improvement was about 75% (Figures 24.9A and B).

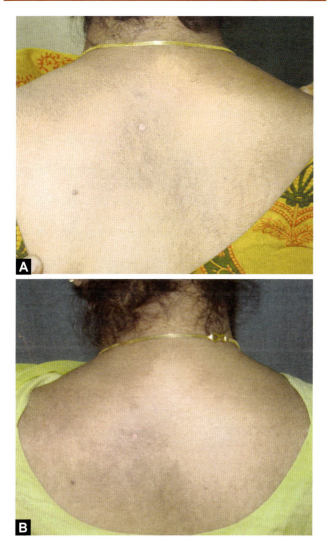

Figs 24.9A and B Macular amyloidosis treated with salicylic acid peels followed by combination peels of glycolic acid kojic acid and hydroquinone

Case 10

Niti Khunger

PROBLEM

- Photoaging
- Type V skin, dermatosis papulosa nigra (DPN) with melasma.

SOLUTION

Priming: Priming is started with sunscreen combined with hydroquinone 4% in the morning (Brite cream) and combination glycolic acid 10%, kojic acid 2%, hydroquinone 2% (Glyaha-Koj cream®), applied for 1 hour in the evening. When it is well tolerated, tretinoin cream 0.025% is started after 1 week, applied for 1 hour in the night. DPN lesions are treated with radiofrequency, cut coagulate mode.

Peeling: After 2 weeks, chemical peeling with salicylic acid 30%, every 2 weeks is done, to smoothen the skin and reduce pigmentation. Then sequential peeling with glycolic acid 35 to 70% for 2 minutes, followed by salicylic acid 30%. It is repeated every 2 weeks, increasing duration and strength of glycolic acid gradually. Spot 15% TCA peel to persistent areas (Figures 24.10A and B).

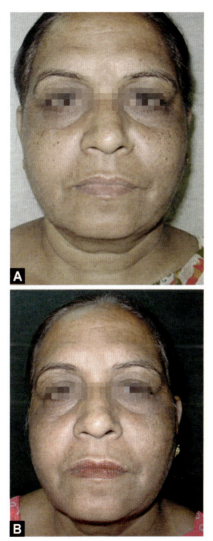

Figs 24.10A and B DPN lesions treated with radiofrequency followed by salicylic acid peels

Case 11

Jaishree Sharad

PROBLEM

A 26-year-old girl, type 4 skin, with acne and hyperpigmentation due to excoriation and grade 1 scars. She was married and planning to conceive in the next few months. Hence, no oral medications were given (Figures 24.11A and B).

SOLUTION

Topical regime given was Cetaphil® cleansing lotion and topical clindamycin gel 1% and sunscreen gel. Chemical peels were initiated with 3 sessions of 20% salicylic acid and 20% glycolic acid peels sequentially at 2 week intervals. These were followed by 3 sessions of 15% TCA peels. The interval between two subsequent peels was 2 weeks. Her skin cleared up in 3 months.

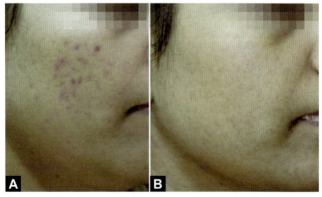

Figs 24.11A and B Acne with pigmentation treated with combination and sequential peels

Case 12

Jaishree Sharad

PROBLEM

A 22-year-old female, type 4 skin with postinflammatory hyperpigmentation after trauma. The duration was three months (Figures 24.12A and B).

SOLUTION

Four sessions of Nomelan® phenol peel were done at 2 week intervals followed by 2 sessions of yellow peel® every 2 weeks. All her pigmentation cleared with phenol peels. Her skin texture smoothened and tone-evened out with the yellow peel.

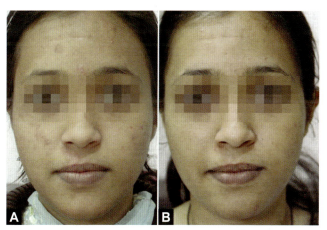

Figs 24.12A and B Postinflammatory hyperpigmentation treated with sequential peels

Case 13

Shenaz Arsiwala

PROBLEM

A 29-year-old female patient, skin type 4, with adult acne presenting with papular and inflammatory lesions on chin, cheeks and persistent lesions on nasolabial folds along with marked panfacial seborrhea. On hormonal evaluation, there was no polycystic ovarian syndrome or adrenal hyperfunction. Patient wished to avoid oral isotretinoin and hormonal therapy (Figures 24.13A and B).

SOLUTION

She was started on oral azithromycin 500 mg daily, three days a week, topical adapalene 0.1% and benzoyl peroxide 2.5% with partial response. Chemical peels added at 8 weeks

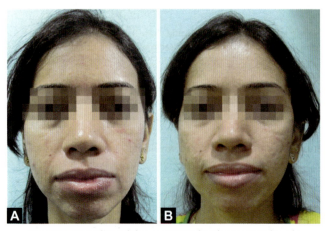

Figs 24.13A and B Adult acne treated with sequential peels

after priming with 10% glycolic acid cream and gel based broadspectrum sunscreen. Peel choice was 30% salicylic acid and 20% mandelic acid peel done sequentially in same sitting for 4 sessions, at fortnightly intervals. There was reduction in existing inflammatory and papular acne, fewer number of new acne lesions, reduction in postacne erythematous scars and marked improvement in seborrhea and skin texture after 4 sessions.

Further therapies would include maintenance with topical adapalene and benzoyl peroxide with sunscreens and plan for acne scar intervention with fractional ablative lasers with subcision.

Case 14

Shenaz Arsiwala

PROBLEM

A 24-year-old female patient presented with a postinflammatory hyperpigmented linear patch on the left zygomatic area extending on lateral periorbital rim sustained after burns with hair iron. She also had mild acne with postinflammatory erythematous macules (Figures 24.14A and B).

SOLUTION

After adequate counseling, she was started on topical hydroquinone 2% with broadspectrum sunscreen and topical adapalene for acne. There was partial response in pigment reduction. After above priming regimen patient was started on combination chemical peels using 20% blend of salicylic and glycolic acid with retinol, kojic acid and vitamin C enhancers added in the above peel cocktail.

Total clearance of linear pigment was obtained in 3 sessions of this peeling therapy done every 2 weeks. Reduction

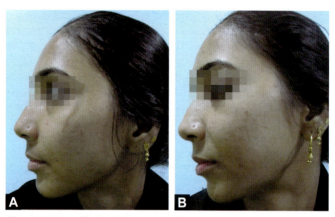

Figs 24.14A and B Postinflammatory hyperpigmentation treated with combination peels

in mild acne as well as postacne macules and texture was also visible.

Further therapies include continuation of topical adapalene and sunscreens along with topical kojic acid as maintenance.

Case 15

Niti Khunger

PROBLEM

A 22-year-old female type 5 skin complained of persisting bluish-gray hyperpigmentation for 3 years. Biopsy showed lichen planus pigmentosus (Figures 24.15A and B).

SOLUTION

Topical priming regimen given was sunscreen with 2% kojic acid and triple combination cream containing tretinoin 0.025%, Fluocinolone acetonide 0.5% and hydroquinone 2% for 4 weeks. This was followed by sequential chemical peels, 20% salicylic acid followed by combination peel containing glycolic acid 20%, kojic acid for 6 peels at 2 week intervals. After a gap of two months, chemical peel was restarted with sequential peel 30% salicylic acid followed by 25% TCA peel for 8 peels at 2 week intervals. Marked improvement was observed at 18 months. There was a mild recurrence after 6 months. Chemical peels were maintained once a month, with a maintenance regime of topical sunscreen and kojic acid and glycolic acid along with tretinoin 0.025%.

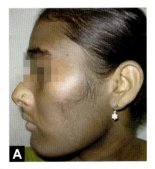 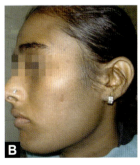

Figs 24.15A and B Dermal pigmentation due to lichen planus treated with combination and sequential peels

25

Ten Golden Rules for Perfect Peeling

Niti Khunger

Rule 1: Counseling Like a Professional

- First visit is most important. Give adequate time.
- Do not pressurize. Do not overload with information. Discuss down time involved and schedule accordingly.
- Establish an expectation alignment. If necessary, call again for counseling. Underplay results without discouraging. Discuss possible complications.

Rule 2: Adequate Priming

- Priming should be done at least 2 to 4 weeks prior to peeling. Examine healed injuries and knuckles. If they are hyperpigmented be cautious. Prime for 4 to 6 weeks.
- Give clear instructions. Use of soaps, facewash, moisturizers and make up should be discussed.
- Sunscreens, glycolic acid, retinoids, hypopigmenting agents should be chosen according to skin type.

Rule 3: Choosing the Right Peel

- *Acne, oily thick skin, scars:* Salicylic acid, trichloroacetic acid (TCA), glycolic acid

- *Dark skin:* Low strength glycolic, salicylic acid, mandelic acid, kojic acid, TCA, gradually titrate strength upwards. Avoid medium and deep peels.
- *Thin, dry, mature sensitive skin:* Lactic acid, mandelic acid, low strength glycolic acid, low strength combination peels.

Rule 4: When not to Peel

- Uncooperative patient. Learn to recognize obsessive, difficult, fussy, careless patients. Refuse outright, unrealistic patients. Be patient but firm. Do not let them bully you or your staff.
- Just before important events and vacations.
- Skin red, burning, incomplete healing.

Rule 5: Applying the Peel

- Degrease gently. Do not rub and scrub.
- Apply uniformly. Look for hotspots. Do not leave the room till peeling is completed.
- For localized lesions do spot peels. Feather at the edges.

Rule 6: Postpeel Care

- Sunscreens, moisturizers, till the skin is peeling. Warn against picking or peeling the skin.
- Restart priming agents. Avoid new agents. Emphasize on regular topical treatment.
- Steroids for excess redness, swelling or burning. Reduce inflammation quickly to prevent postinflammatory hyperpigmentation (PIH).

Rule 7: Detecting Complications Early

- Assess high-risk patients regularly.
- Educate patient to look for warning signs like redness, crusting, pain, infection.

- *Impending complications:* Treat early, treat hard, treat aggressively. If complications occur, do not panic. Admit the complication, give support and tide over the event with a lot of hand-holding.

Rule 8: Combining Peels

- Combine low strength peels to increase efficacy without increasing risk, in high-risk patients.
- Mix and match peels segmentally and sequentially for optimum results.
- Individualize treatment by combining different procedures.

Rule 9: Repeating Peels

- Repeat superficial peels every 2 to 3 weeks for 3 months, then monthly for 6 months. Depending on response, repeat thereafter.
- Repeat medium peels after 3 to 6 months and deep peels after 1 year, if required. Better to underpeel than overpeel.
- Emphasize that maintenance topical treatment is essential.

Rule 10: Do not be Jack of all Peels and Master of None

- Use selected trusted brands. Do not experiment frequently.
- Do not interchange brands in the same patient, even if they are of the same agent and concentration.
- Gain long-term experience and mastery over your peeling agents.

Chemical peels are effective, safe, simple and inexpensive multimodality tools to enhance cosmetic practice in all skin types, all over the world. Newer advances in peels and peel procedures have ensured that peels hold an important place in esthetic procedures despite the onslaught of lasers and other modalities. Treatment can be tailored to individual needs and it is far easier to acquire and maintain ten different peels than three different lasers.

Appendices

Appendix I

Terminology in Chemical Peeling

Chemical peeling: Chemexfoliation or controlled partial thickness injury to the skin by application of a chemical agent at a predetermined concentration, to achieve a desired depth of necrosis.

Acid: Those substances that give hydrogen ions when dissolved in water. Aqueous solutions at 25° with a pH less than seven are considered acidic.

pH: Measure of the acidity or alkalinity of a solution. Negative logarithm of base 10 of hydrogen ion concentration.

pKa: The pH at which the level of free acid is same as the level of the salt of the substance. Negative logarithm of base 10 of dissociation constant of an acid. The less the pKa the stronger the acid.

Priming: Pretreatment with topical agents applied for few weeks before the actual commencement of chemical peeling with the goal of thinning the stratum corneum, enhancing uniform penetration of active agents, decreasing postoperative side effects and complication such as pregnancy-induced hypertension (PIH) and reducing the healing time.

Priming agents: Topical agents used in priming, e.g. tretinoin, hydroquinone, glycolic acid.

α-hydroxy acids (AHAs)—fruit acids: Group of organic carboxylic acids with hydroxy group in alpha position.

Frosting: Change in color of skin to white which represents the end stage of chemical peeling and occurs due to keratin agglutination, seen with TCA, phenol, etc.

Pseudofrosting: White frosting due to crystallization of acid seen with salicylic acid.

Contact time: Duration of the chemical peel after which neutralization is performed.

Neutralization: Critical step performed once the proper depth of peel has been achieved to neutralize the acid using cold water, bicarbonate spray, etc. It is used mainly for α-hydroxy acids.

End point: The point when the peel is terminated.

Very superficial peel: Exfoliation of the stratum corneum, without any epidermal necrosis.

Superficial peel: Destruction of the full epidermis, up to the basal layer.

Medium peel: Destruction of the epidermis, papillary dermis up to the upper one-third of the reticular dermis.

Deep peel: Necrosis of the entire epidermis and papillary dermis, with inflammation extending to the mid-reticular dermis.

Spot peels and regional peels: Chemical peeling over a localized affected area.

Combination peels: Combination of two or more different peeling agents in a single formulation.

Sequential peels: Chemical peels using more than one peel at a time in a sequential manner as they may not be compatible in a single formulation for deeper penetration and multimodal action.

Segmental peels: Using different peels in different cosmetic units, at the same session.

Switch peels: Peels are changed serially in different peeling sessions.

Chemical reconstruction of skin scars (CROSS): Used to treat depressed icepick scars by utilizing high strength TCA.

Appendix II

Consent Form

Mr/Ms ——————————————————————————

Address ——————————————————————————

City——————————————————————————————

Tel Nos. (R) ————(O) ———— (Mobile) ————

Name of the Procedure: Chemical Peels

I ———————————————give consent to the treatment known as chemical peel. I have been explained the type of treatment, procedure, outcome of treatment, likely risks and complications that can arise and time taken for recovery of normal skin in a language I understand. I have been advised that though good results are expected, they cannot be guaranteed. I understand that multiple sessions may be needed for satisfactory results and even after the final procedure, maintenance treatment may be essential to maintain results and recurrences may occur. I have had an opportunity to ask questions and discuss alternative treatments.

I also know that the procedure will be performed by Dr ——— or an assistant ——————————— who is qualified to perform this procedure. I also give consent that during the procedure, if anything goes wrong I may be given any emergency treatment best suitable to me. I agree to follow all instructions given to me by the doctor.

I have carefully read and understood all information provided in this form and under fully conscious mind, I hereby give my written consent for the said procedure with its risks involved. I also give consent for medical photographs.

Signature of patient/Thumb impression: —————————

Signature of Parents/Guardian (for Minors) ————————

Date: —————— Place: ——————————————

Witness:

Name —————— Signature ————— Date ———

Appendix III

Patient Handouts

Name:
Age/Sex:
Doctor's Address and contact no:
Schedule of peels:

Prepeel Instructions

Once you have decided to undergo chemical peels, you must follow instructions carefully:

1. Avoid sun exposure as far as possible, particularly between 10 am–4 pm. Use physical measures like umbrella, broad-brim hat and cover with clothes, when going out for prolonged periods.

2. Use sunscreens daily as advised. Apply 20 to 30 minutes before going out so that it has time to bond with the skin. Use an adequate amount, little more than half a teaspoon (3 ml) each to the face, neck and forearm. It is better to apply more sunscreen with lower sun protection factor (SPF) than very little sunscreen with higher SPF. Use even on a cloudy day as UV light is still present. Reapply after swimming for more than 40 minutes and after 2 hours while sweating. Never forget your sunscreen when going for a vacation. Always apply at beaches due to increased reflection from the sand and water and at hill stations because of increased exposure to UV light at high altitudes.

3. Clean your face with the cleanser prescribed according to your skin type.

4. You have informed your doctor about all allergies, skin diseases like atopic dermatitis, seborrheic dermatitis, eczemas, photodermatitis and herpes that you have suffered and medications, especially pain killers, isotretinoin, diuretics,

antidiabetics and antihypertensives that you are taking. If there is any additional information please inform before the peel.

5. Do not bleach, wax, scrub, massage or use loofahs, sponges, depilatories or scrubs 1 week before the peel.

6. Stop retinoids 1 week before the peel and resume when peeling is complete.

7. Do not schedule any important event or vacation for at least 1 to 5 days after a superficial peel and 7 to 10 days after a medium depth peel.

8. On the day of the peel, come with a clean face and no make-up. Men should avoid shaving on the day of the peel and not use cologne or after shave. Carry your sunscreen with you.

9. Remove your contact lenses before the peel.

Prepeel	Name	Strength	Time
a. Sunscreen			
b. Retinoid			
c. Hydroquinone			
d. Glycolic acid			
e. Any other			
f. Antiviral			

Day of the Peel

1. Sign consent form
2. Have photographs taken
3. Wash the face
4. Remove contact lenses

Postpeel Instructions

1. Peeling will be obvious, particularly after the first peel and it may take up to 1 week for the skin to return to normal. Stinging, burning, itching, tightness and redness

may occur. The skin may look darker, do not get alarmed. Sometimes peeling is not obvious, but the peel will still act.

2. Use ice compresses every 15 minutes, after the peel, till burning subsides.

3. Use the sunscreen in the morning and apply calamine lotion in a moisturizing base for stinging sensation.

4. Use moisturizer for feeling of tightness as frequently as desired, so that you are comfortable, till the skin returns to normal.

5. Wash gently and use a cleanser as advised. Do not rub or use any scrubs or abrasive agents.

6. *Most important:* Do not pick, peel, scratch, rub or scrub the skin.

7. Report immediately, if you see crusts, oozing, pus formation, blisters, excessive redness, swelling, burning or pain.

8. Start the maintenance regimen given, when the skin returns to normal.

	Name	Strength	Time
a. Sunscreen			
b. Moisturizer			
c. Calamine lotion			
d. Soap/cleanser			
e. Maintenance regimen			
f. Any other			

Appendix IV

Ethical Aspects of Chemical Peels

Aesthetic or cosmetic surgery is performed to improve physical appearances in the absence of a significant pathology. Today, dermatosurgeons practice in an increasingly complex health care environment that is characterized by a variety of challenging influences. The growing influence of the media on consumers and its erroneous portrayal of cosmetic surgery, particularly chemical peels, as being so simple that it can be performed outside a physician's office or by a non-physician has led to demanding and persistent patients seeking perfection. Many patients regard aesthetic surgery as a panacea for their personal and relationship difficulties. Some may also be suffering from an underlying body dysmorphic disorder (BDD), which is a psychiatric syndrome, characterized by an obsession with a non-existent or minimal cosmetic "defect" associated with persistent attempts to have the defect corrected. The fussy patient with imagined or minor complaints is potential problem patients and should be approached with care.

Proper selection of patient, adequate counseling, obtaining informed consent and choosing the right peel for the right patient are the cornerstones for ethical practice. The physician must be guided by sound ethical principles rather than commercial interests.

The three basic principles of ethical practice are:

1. Respect for patient autonomy
2. Beneficience
3. Non-maleficence

Another area of growing concern is the use of non-approved agents and appropriate delegation of procedures to trained, qualified medical staff under direct, on-site supervision. The physician must directly supervise the non-physician office personnel, should be physically present on-site, immediately available, and able to respond promptly to any problem that may occur while the procedure is being performed. It is the physician's obligation to ensure that the non-physician office personnel possess the proper training in cutaneous medicine and are well aware of the indications for the procedure, and the pre- and postoperative care involved, in order to protect the best interests and welfare of each patient.

In today's demanding world of interventional procedures to obtain quick and perfect results, ethical practice of cosmetic surgery is becoming more and more difficult. The treating physician should use experience and judgment to establish ethical practice, while at the same time, avoid being overcautious and having a negative approach, to minimize potential medicolegal liabilities.

Index

Page numbers followed by *f* refer to figure and *t* refer to table